Five Key Strategies to

Gain Control Over Your Psoriasis

A science-based treatment plan using lifestyle & intuitive eating

By Caylee Clay, RDN, CDN, CYT

First Edition

ISBN-13: 978-1-7351504-1-3

Cover design by: Caylee Clay
Formatting by Polgarus Studio
Printed in the United States of America

This book is for educational purposes only. While the author has used their best efforts in preparing this book, no representations or warranties are made with respect to the accuracy or completeness of the contents of this book and specifically disclaims any implied warranties of merchantability or fitness for a particular purpose. No warranty may be created or extended by sales representatives or written sales materials. The advice and strategies contained herein may not be suitable for your situation, and do not substitute, or constitute, professional care by a medical provider. You should consult with a professional where appropriate. The author shall not be liable for any loss of profit or any other commercial damages, including but not limited to special, incidental, consequential, or other damages.

The information contained in this book is not intended to serve as a replacement for professional medical advice. Any use of the information in this book is at the reader's discretion. The author specifically disclaims any and all liability arising directly or indirectly from the use or application of any information contained in this book. Please work with a team of healthcare providers such as a dietitian nutritionist, therapist, medical doctor, and/or other relevant providers to best understand how this information may apply to your individual situation and medical condition(s). Please note that new research is being published daily and best practices may later be redefined as new information becomes available.

To my wonderful parents, brother, and partner

who never doubted my vision

and always supported my dreams.

Contents

△ △ △ △

FOREWORD

"Illness provides us with an invitation for self-transformation, an opportunity to change our way of thinking, feeling, eating and in general caring for ourselves and our lives."

— Vasant Lad, BAMS MASc,
founder of the Ayurvedic Institute and author of
The Complete Book of Ayurvedic Home Remedies

△ △ △ △

Psoriasis is a complex condition that impacts the body at many different levels. For anyone who is struggling with psoriasis and is seeking a more holistic approach to coping with symptoms, this is the book for you! *Gain Control Over Your Psoriasis* provides straightforward, simple, and actionable steps that you can take to help you better manage your symptoms.

I am a biologist, wellness consultant, and lifestyle educator who helps individuals throughout the world take control of their well-being. For a condition that can seem to be unmanageable at times, nutrition and lifestyle can play critical roles in helping you improve your psoriasis. In moments of reflection, it's important to become aware of how you feel and mindful of your symptoms. Since Caylee and I often discuss psoriasis research, I was so happy to hear that she was writing this book! Caylee is so passionate about not only sharing her psoriasis journey with others, but also explaining nutritional research. This book brings awareness to the many diet and lifestyle factors that may be impacting your particular condition.

As a biologist, I have written extensively on the topic of psoriasis. I have informed dermatologists and other healthcare professionals about the comorbidities associated with psoriasis and overall quality of life. Yet, I realized that although healthcare professionals are continuously receiving up-to-date information on the pharmaceutical drugs that treat psoriasis, most are not aware of the latest research regarding psoriasis from a nutritional standpoint. However, I know that not everyone has access to the latest nutritional studies published in the scientific and medical literature, or the time to sort through all the data. That's where this book comes in. It helps to bridge this knowledge gap by providing an evidence-based and comprehensive overview of psoriasis from a diet and lifestyle perspective.

Caylee is not only a registered dietitian nutritionist, but has struggled with psoriasis herself! Therefore, she offers a unique perspective on psoriasis management by combining her personal and professional experience. Caylee knows what it's like to try to make sense of flare-ups, and by becoming more aware of her symptoms and triggers, she has successfully been able to tame her psoriasis from within. And now, she wants to share with you her best practices through an evidence-based approach to help you with your psoriasis journey.

Gain Control Over Your Psoriasis offers a more holistic approach to managing psoriasis from all different standpoints. As the saying goes, "Let food be thy medicine." But as a psoriasis sufferer, how do you know which foods may help make your condition more manageable? As a dietitian nutritionist, Caylee profoundly understands the role that eating patterns play in psoriasis and educates others on making better food choices, recommends dietary guidelines, and indicates which potential food sensitivities to consider. Although diet and lifestyle vary from one person to another, this book offers proactive approaches to addressing several food and lifestyle triggers. It provides you with options so that you are better informed to make educated decisions for your overall health. And when you are equipped with the right tools, you have the power to manage your psoriasis better!

Be informed! Be well!

Nicole Marie Benvin, Ph.D.
Biologist, Wellness Consultant, and Lifestyle Educator

△ △ △ △

Introduction

"The natural healing force within each of us is the greatest force in getting well."

— Hippocrates,
ancient physician & father of modern medicine

△ △ △ △

Living with psoriasis is no small feat. There is plenty of pain and suffering – both physical and emotional – wrapped up in this disease state. The goal of this book is to help you gain an understanding of what triggers, as well as what improves, your psoriasis so that you can feel more in control of your symptoms and pain levels and therefore, your life. This book will harness the power of the foods you eat and lifestyle you live to promote the healing process, which ultimately will help you to manage your psoriasis better with less pain. This approach is based in science and personalized. It also does not utilize unsustainable excessive dietary restrictions nor does it require or even recommend weight loss. Instead of prescribing a diet, in this book you will find information on how to make peace with both the food you eat and your psoriasis. In fact, you will gain the most from this book if you have already rejected the diet mentality entirely, and accepted that weight is not a true indicator of health status. As you read along, you will be encouraged to listen to your body to identify healing and harmful foods, and will learn how to include both in your life in a balance that leans towards self-healing. The recommendations in the book are gentle, depend on self-compassion, and prioritize reducing your pain and suffering. **The goal is to identify exactly what helps and hurts your psoriasis, so ultimately you spend much less time thinking about psoriasis and food and can instead focus on living your best life.**

As someone who suffered from this miserable condition myself – but has experienced complete remission, thanks to the info in this book! – I know firsthand that one of the most frustrating aspects of having psoriasis can be the feeling that your flare-ups and healing phases are random and outside of your control. I set out to attempt to identify all of my psoriasis triggers, so I could at least understand what was causing my flare-ups instead of feeling helpless and hopeless. This book is the compilation of the several years of research I put into this topic.

Psoriasis is often thought of as just a problem with the skin, but the truth is that psoriasis is more than simply a skin condition: psoriasis is also an autoimmune disease. Autoimmune diseases arise when the immune system malfunctions and launches an inflammatory attack, in this case affecting our skin cells.[1] This immunological attack can also spread to our joint cells, as between 18 - 42% of people with psoriasis will also develop psoriatic arthritis.[2] Plus, it's important to note that about 25% of people with one autoimmune disease go on to develop additional autoimmune diseases.[3] Therefore, it's best to understand and treat psoriasis through the lens of the immune system, instead of simply the skin. Any treatments that only address the skin will simply serve as a mask for the symptoms of psoriasis, and will not address the root causes.

To best manage psoriasis, we need to understand more about the immune system. The immune system is a collection of organs, cells, and natural chemicals that defends our bodies against infection, disease, and toxins. About 70% of our entire immune system resides in our gut,[4] meaning that our gut health and the food we eat can have a large impact on whether our psoriasis improves or gets worse. Therefore, it's of paramount importance to consume foods that optimize gut health, lower inflammation, and support immune health. There is no one-size-fits-all psoriasis "diet" or eating pattern – in fact, while one way of eating may improve the psoriasis of some, others may find no benefit to their psoriasis by eating the same way. It is clear that different foods may be aggravating or beneficial to different people. It is essential to identify individual dietary triggers instead of offering blanket suggestions to all psoriasis sufferers. However, it's also important that we always leave room to enjoy our favorite foods, even if they trigger our psoriasis! This is a delicate but critical balance. The gentlest and most holistic way to identify individual dietary triggers while still being "allowed" to consume our favorite foods is by using a method called "intuitive eating," which will be explained in depth later on. Additionally, how we live our lives – our lifestyle – can either support or hinder our healing process.

My personal journey of healing my own psoriasis has been a long and winding path, but along the way I have learned an incredible wealth of techniques, strategies, and coping mechanisms to help reduce psoriasis. Not only has my personal journey greatly augmented my understanding of psoriasis, but my professional role as a dietitian nutritionist has led me to the conclusion that the role of the gut is highly underappreciated and underutilized in the treatment of psoriasis. As a medical professional, I believe that the complex interplay between our intestinal health, microbiome, genetics, eating patterns, lifestyle, environment, and immune system will one day provide a scientific explanation for how and why psoriasis develops, plus what we can do to reduce psoriasis or possibly even put it into remission reliably. In the process of writing this book, my psoriasis finally went into complete remission for the first time in 6.5 years! My passion is to share all of this knowledge with you and at minimum reduce your psoriasis, if not put it completely into remission, too.

In this book, you will gain many tools to support your body in healing itself. You will learn how to avoid several different types of intestinal injuries that excessively burden your immune system, and how to deal with it when those injuries do, inevitably, occur. You will develop an understanding of how to optimize your intestinal health and, by extension, your immune health. You will learn about the microscopic world of critters that live in and on you called the microbiome, and how they influence your psoriasis plus what you can do to support the health-giving microbes. You will explore the genetic relationships associated with psoriasis and related health concerns, and how to reduce their negative health effects. You will discover strategies that you can use for a lifetime to ease the pain and distress caused by psoriasis. You will learn how to trust your own body and experiences to guide your healing journey, using concepts like intuitive eating. You will be encouraged to reconnect with your body and bodily symptoms (something that can be quite scary for those of us who suffer from the chronic pain of living with psoriasis!) in order to facilitate the healing process.

This book contains a lot of information. It does take a dedicated person to implement these suggestions to experience the full benefits. If at any point you find that it is too overwhelming, please do note that I am available for one-on-one appointments. I offer in-person appointments for those who are able to travel to my offices in New York City, and I also offer virtual and phone appointments for those who live further away or who prefer to not travel. Please visit my website at www.autoimmuneeats.com to inquire about booking an appointment.

Wishing you ample natural healing, clear answers, and happier living as you continue on your psoriasis journey!

✦ Introduction to My Psoriasis Story ✦

It's hard to say exactly when my psoriasis story begins. Does it begin in late elementary school – perhaps it was 5th grade – when my friends first made fun of me for having red flaking skin around my nose? Does it begin in 10th grade when I had strep throat, which is a significant trigger for psoriasis? The memory of my great aunt buying me exfoliating shower gloves and specifically instructing me to scrub the extra skin off of my elbows? Does it begin with my relatives who were also diagnosed with autoimmune diseases, plus the relatives that (I believe) had undiagnosed autoimmune diseases? I'm not sure. All I really know is that psoriasis became a serious, notable, and unwavering problem in my life in 2012.

Right before then, in the fall of 2011, I was living through something that is extremely common with many psoriasis sufferers: chronic stress. Ironically, I was studying healthcare as a student at New York University, working towards my Bachelors of Science in Nutrition and on my way to becoming a registered dietitian nutritionist. I had two jobs, I was overworked from the rigorous demands of my university classes, I was sleep deprived, and I had already been living in polluted NYC for a few years – plus I was doubling down on breathing in this pollution by biking around the city almost daily. To no surprise, I got sick. I ended up with walking pneumonia, an ear infection, and a vaginal yeast infection. I went to the doctor, and was prescribed antibiotics. And so the health of my intestinal microbiome began to decline.

Then, in the summer of 2012, I was overworked yet again. I had a demanding part-time job plus I was taking summer college classes. Even though I was eating a decent amount of healthy food, I was also eating a decent amount of less healthy foods and plenty of sugar. That summer, I ended up with laryngitis plus a nasty cough, I had several vaginal yeast infections, I was biking through polluted NYC streets regularly, and also moved apartments. During the 2012 fall semester, I was getting increasingly ill. Not only did I have psoriasis, but I also had joint pains that at certain times became excruciating (I have never been diagnosed with psoriatic arthritis, but have little doubt that I would have been at this time if I had known to go to a rheumatologist). I was losing weight without trying or wanting to. I remember in the winter of 2012 - 2013, I was in such pain that the only place I could get some sleep was on a cold, hard, wooden floor – for whatever reason, this eased my joint pain just enough so I could finally fall asleep. I didn't seek medical attention because I didn't know how to use my health insurance (which is a whole other topic of discussion for another time), and felt too overwhelmed by my college studies to find a healthcare provider who could maybe help me – an ironic mistake that I will only make once!

I was about to hold off on my last semester of college until, by chance, I tried going gluten-free. Within a few weeks, my joint pain greatly improved and I could go back to sleeping in my bed. My psoriasis cleared completely. The only concern was that my hips flared up with this incredibly itchy rash – so itchy I simply could not stop itching until I bled, however the whole rest of my body felt better. Even though this rash was very alarming, I knew I couldn't go back to eating gluten. I later learned that what I was experiencing is colloquially known as "Candida die-off," known in the medical community as the Jarisch-Herxheimer reaction (more on this in the Sugar section). Over the next several months, I started putting back on some much needed weight. I went from scarily sick to thriving in a few short months, and finished my college degree with flying colors.

A common saying in the medical field is that "genetics loads the gun, but the environment pulls the trigger," and I find this to be very accurate for those of us with psoriasis. When I first started developing notable psoriasis, the environmental triggers of chronic stress, high sugar intake, lack of sleep, and poor air quality were all present and set off the genetic gun of psoriasis. The autoimmune genes I now know I inherited from my family were awakened. Around this time, my psoriasis would come and go, and I was actually able to put my psoriasis and joint pain into complete remission by avoiding consuming gluten. That would soon change.

Then came February 2014. This was the last time I took a round of antibiotics. I had a kidney infection. Soon after those antibiotics were finished, my psoriasis flared up like never before. Although I am extremely thankful to have two fully functioning kidneys now, the damage was done elsewhere. It has taken me 6.5 years since those antibiotics to finally put my psoriasis back into remission. I later learned that not only can antibiotics disrupt what before was a healthy microbiome, but since they kill off bacteria in large quantities, they leave your intestines open to opportunistic fungal infections. By 2015, I was finally officially a dietitian nutritionist – and one with increasing psoriasis.

The next year, in 2016, I was sitting in my office at work between appointments with my nutrition clients and staring at the psoriasis patches on my elbows in frustration. What was causing my skin to behave like this? Why was this happening to me? What could I do to improve it? I rested my elbow on the desk and tried to hold my head up with my empty palm – but jerked back from the pain of putting pressure on my raw psoriatic elbow. I had 4 chronic patches of psoriasis between my two elbows, 2 more chronic patches on my ankles, plus random patches that would come and go seemingly at their own will. What was going on?

In 2018, I finally scheduled an appointment with a dermatologist to get a diagnosis that I already knew I had: psoriasis. The doctor was kind, but not too helpful – she offered me a steroid cream. I said thanks, but no thanks. She politely asked why I wouldn't use the medication. I told her that no steroid cream will fix the root problem of what's actually causing my psoriasis – it just masks the symptoms. She reminded me that there's "no cure" for psoriasis. Anyone else tired of hearing that same line over and over?

Flash forward to 2020. I went from having 6 chronic, painful patches of psoriasis plus various flare-ups all over my body, to now being in complete remission! I achieved this entirely by changing the foods I eat and my lifestyle. During the years leading up to my remission, I painstakingly identified which triggers flared up my psoriasis and also discovered many strategies to heal myself quicker and quicker after a flare-up. For a few years, I reached a point where I understood my triggers so well that I could choose to have a flare-up, which was an incredible reprieve from hoping and praying against all odds that my skin would stay calm. To now be in complete remission is just icing on the proverbial cake (which sadly I can only eat sparingly due to the gluten and sugar – but more on that later!)

Years of personal experience, countless hours of research, a background in health sciences, plus working with psoriatic clients in my nutrition private practice have led me to intimately understand how eating patterns deeply influence psoriasis severity. It is my immense pleasure (and possibly life's calling) to collect this information into one central place so that others such as yourself may benefit from my findings and discover true relief from your psoriasis. I hope you gain as much healing, comfort, and self-awareness as I have from the information in this book.

△ △ △ △

The Game Plan

"There is no one size fits all. There is no magic diet, pill, or plan. We eat. We eat to nourish. We eat to celebrate. We eat to socialize. The only rule is there are no rules. There is room for everyone here."

— Christyna Johnson, MS, RDN, LD
Non-Diet Registered Dietitian

△ △ △ △

This book is organized into five main strategies for reducing and managing your psoriasis, each filled with recommendations based on scientific research as well as my own personal and professional experiences. **It is my goal to clearly explain the recommendations that research supports in plain English, while separating out the more in-depth scientific aspects followed by my own experiences, so you can easily identify the information that is most relevant to you and your level of interest.** While I suggest utilizing these five main strategies in order, you can explore these strategies in any order (however, the More on the Science and My Psoriasis Story sections do build on each other chronologically, so it may be best to read those sections in order). To gain maximum benefit, you will need to revisit most of the strategies multiple times and reimplement the various recommendations over time as the needs of your psoriasis change and you gain a deeper understanding of your triggers.

While the food we eat can have a profound effect on the

severity of our psoriasis, it is of utmost importance to understand that people with autoimmune diseases are at an increased risk for developing eating disorders.[1,2,3] Eating disorders are extremely serious medical conditions with a low recovery rate and a high death rate.[4,5,6] Eating disorders are characterized by irregular eating habits, severe distress or concern about body weight or shape, and may include inadequate or excessive food intake. The most common forms of eating disorders include anorexia nervosa, bulimia nervosa, and binge eating disorder. Eating disorders are classified as a mental illness.[7]

I commonly see disordered eating habits, behaviors, and thought processes in my clients with autoimmune diseases at my nutrition private practice. As a result, I strongly urge against using severe food restrictions as an attempt to manage your psoriasis. In general, I would consider "severe" as trying to maintain greater than 2 - 3 food restrictions at a time. See the Eating Attitudes Test (EAT) section in the Appendix if you would like to complete an individual assessment. Additionally, please note that in this book I try to refrain from using the word "diet" as much as possible, since this word is now primarily defined as a highly restrictive eating pattern that we have to force onto ourselves and likely cannot maintain. Instead of using this potentially triggering word, you will see terms such as "eating pattern" or "the food we eat" to refer to the kinds of food that we normally, regularly, and habitually eat – and does *not* refer to a highly restrictive way of eating.

With this knowledge of the increased risk of eating disorders in our psoriasis community, I made the very deliberate decision to align the recommendations in this book as much as possible with the 10 principles of intuitive eating. The intuitive eating movement has been largely adopted by dietitian nutritionists who specialize in eating disorder treatment, as research demonstrates that intuitive eating is associated with a lower risk of eating disorders.[8] Psoriasis sufferers are also at greater risk for developing cardiovascular disease,[9,10] and intuitive eating can help reduce our risk of this disease as well. The intuitive eating approach absolutely avoids all "diets" and is instead anti-diet. To utilize intuitive eating, it is necessary to reject this diet mentality, plus any dreams of an "ideal" weight or body shape or size that may be attached to it. Since eating disorders may develop as a way to attempt to control body size, rejecting dieting and dreams of unrealistic weight loss necessarily go hand-in-hand. This means that, over time, your weight will stabilize, which is healthier for your cardiovascular system. People whose weight repeatedly goes up and down – called "weight cycling" or "yo-yo dieting" – have TWICE the normal risk of dying from heart disease.[11]

Especially if you are considered "overweight," you may have heard from healthcare providers that your psoriasis will improve if you lose weight. I'm here to respectfully disagree with that antiquated and incorrect thought. The entirety of the info in this book is aimed at actually reducing your psoriasis and the associated pain, not at changing your body size or shape. This concept is called Health at Every Size (HAES). HAES argues that weight loss is prescribed as a panacea and is not nearly as health-producing as we once thought, and instead harms individuals across the size spectrum with stigmatization plus perpetuates our "cultural obsession with weight loss and thinness."[12] HAES and intuitive eating are paradigms that can support healing and longevity in the psoriasis community in many ways.

Psoriasis is a chronic disease, and probably just about every healthcare practitioner you've ever seen has been quick to remind you that there is no "cure" for psoriasis. As someone who has experienced remission with my own psoriasis, I staunchly feel that this belief should be fiercely questioned and debated. There are many case studies and individual reports in support groups of folks whose psoriasis has gone into remission and has been, effectively, "cured." However, in the same vein, you should expect that naturally reducing your psoriasis to be a lengthy process. Additionally, it may be the simple truth that some of us will have to live with psoriasis to some degree for the rest of our lifetimes. While some of us may never completely recover from our psoriasis, there is still so much that can be done to reduce the amount of psoriasis we have and to lessen its negative effects on our lives. To objectively measure your psoriasis severity, use the Calculate Psoriasis Area and Severity Index (PASI) in the Appendix. Some of the strategies in the book may quickly offer relief in a few hours or days, while others may take a few weeks or months before you start to see the benefit. It may take years to realize the full potential benefits of these strategies.

While I expect that you begin to see benefits from these strategies quickly, please also keep in mind that backtracking is a natural part of the process of changing your habits. You will make a healthy change and then go backwards. Your psoriasis will improve and then it will flare up again. You will move forward and then lose ground. You will make mistakes, sometimes by accident and other times knowingly. Backtracking is perfectly normal, absolutely natural, and completely fine. It's actually an integral part of the process. When you find strategies that help improve your psoriasis and then have trouble sticking to them, that's when you learn how significant those strategies are to your psoriasis management. If you aim for a "two steps forward and one step back" approach where you don't backtrack completely, then eventually you will get to where you want to go with your health. Intuitive eating will help you to make peace with this learning process.

Additionally, it's also very important to know that at times your psoriasis will get worse right before it gets much better. If you try something new for your psoriasis and it changes – especially in a way that it's never changed before – that may actually be a good sign! Stay strong while making new changes and stay the course even when it seems like things might be getting worse, because things might get worse on the way to getting better! Not confusing at all, right? One really great clue as to whether your psoriasis is getting worse on the way to getting better is if your flare-up is *different* from prior flare-ups. Psoriasis formation in a new place, after you've made potentially helpful changes, is a good sign!

While you can use the five key strategies outlined in this book in any order, I do suggest starting with the first strategy, which is to add healing foods to those that you usually eat. Psychologically, this helps set us up for success by viewing food as the nurturing and powerful agent of healing that it is. This gives us the freedom to focus on all the wonderful things we can add to our life to improve it, instead of focusing on what to take away. Additionally, since autoimmune diseases and eating disorders often occur together, this demotes the likelihood of triggering an eating disorder while trying to manage our psoriasis. However, if you are suffering through a particularly nasty flare-up and are desperate for relief, then you will likely find the quickest healing from Strategies #3 and #4, on food sensitivities and foods to reduce. Nevertheless, *a word of warning*: if you decide to jump ahead, then I would suggest that you first honestly assess your risk of developing or triggering an eating disorder by working with these strategies, and/or work closely with healthcare providers such as a dietitian nutritionist and psychologist trained in eating disorders to continually help you assess this risk. Please see the Eating Attitudes Test (EAT) section of the appendix to understand if disordered eating or an eating disorder may be present.

The five key strategies outlined in this book are backed by research and have specific physiological objectives. One of the main objectives is to reduce intestinal injuries. Since about 70% of our immune system lies within our digestive system,[13] maintaining digestive health is intimately connected to our immune health. Sustaining intestinal injuries – such as consuming a food you are sensitive to, physically damaging your intestinal tract, or creating an environment that harms your intestinal tract – are hard on your immune system, and therefore, hard on your autoimmune disease. While food can be the cause of intestinal injuries, food is also crucial in helping us heal from these injuries by providing essential nutrients. Figuring out how to optimize our eating patterns in order to minimize these types of intestinal injuries and reduce the load on our immune system is a large part of the journey towards naturally reducing our psoriasis.

Another main objective is to demote the expression of the genes correlated with psoriasis. The study of genetics has taught us that just because we have a certain gene doesn't mean that gene will necessarily get "turned on" and be expressed, and instead the environment we live in heavily influences gene expression. The popular medical saying "genetics loads the gun, but the environment pulls the trigger" is quite apropo here. Additionally, it is possible to "turn off" or regulate gene expression,[14] so this book also aims to create an exterior as well as interior environment that encourages our psoriasis genes to turn off, or at least be expressed less. The web of biological, chemical, and environmental components connecting eating patterns and lifestyle to psoriasis is quite extensive and complex.

However, it's also critical to mention that you are not worth less because you have psoriasis. You have the exact same value as any other human being no matter how much psoriasis you have or don't have. Reducing your psoriasis won't make you a better, more worthy, or more moral person. Instead, reducing your psoriasis will reduce your pain and suffering. That is the goal of this book: reducing pain and suffering. Then, you can focus on other things like living your best life without psoriasis constantly hanging over you like an ominous cloud. I hope to illuminate that having psoriasis is not your fault, as you will see how many triggers are outside of our immediate control – such as the declining quality of our food supply, pervasive air pollution, subacute chronic infections, genetics – and play a role in psoriasis development. Yet, we can alter our way of living to address some of these triggers and reduce their impact on our psoriasis, even if we can't change the problem at large. For example, we can reduce the impact that air pollution has on us even if we can't change the total amount of air pollution in our community.

I organized this book so that first you will read about the 10 principles of intuitive eating. The last principle, gentle nutrition, is the one this book relies on most. Next, you will discover foods and nutrients that are recommended to add to your life. The subsequent section covers meal timing and how that relates to intestinal as well as overall metabolic health. Then you will learn about foods that appear to be common food sensitivities for psoriasis sufferers. You may benefit from eliminating one or some of these food groups, but in my personal and professional experience you almost certainly will not need to eliminate more than one. After that, I address foods that likely are irritating your psoriasis, and that you should limit your intake of. Lifestyle considerations will then be discussed. Finally, the topic of weight stigma and being "overweight" in relationship to psoriasis is explored.

Let's begin your healing journey!

△ △ △ △

The 10 Principles of Intuitive Eating

"Remember that diet culture has the mission of selling you a product. A solution to a 'problem.' Health is not a product. It is not a place where you arrive. It is not an item on a check list. It is complex and complicated. And that's okay."

— Christyna Johnson, MS, RDN, LD
Non-Diet Registered Dietitian

△ △ △ △

Intuitive eating is a way of relearning how to eat and restructuring our relationship with food in a way that rejects all strict diets and other forms of dieting. It requires tuning into your own body to identify healing. Intuitive eating allows us to eat anything and everything we want to eat at all times. At first, this license to eat anything and everything may be scary as it may prompt eating experiences that seem "out of control" and feel like "overeating" or "binging," but it's important to go through these experiences so that once you've grown tired of eating anything and everything, you may find that you are now more drawn to focusing on eating foods that make you feel better. **You forever maintain unconditional permission to eat anything and everything whenever you would like to, and should always look to your body to tell you**

what and how it wants to eat. This ultimately builds up trust in your own relationship with food and your body, which is incredibly healing on many levels.

The below 10 principles are meant to be implemented in order. While this book was absolutely written with the intuitive eating paradigm in mind, please note that the strategies provided in this book assume that you are largely competent with the below principles. If you have a history of dieting, disordered eating or eating disorders, and/or have been on the receiving end of fat shaming (such as falsely being told that your psoriasis would improve if you "just" lost weight), then it is highly recommended that you work with an anti-diet dietitian and/or therapist who are aligned with intuitive eating and the Health at Every Size (HAES) movement to help you recover from these traumatic events before utilizing this book for psoriasis relief. While examples of intuitive eating can be found throughout the entire book, in general this book lies within the realm of principle #10: honor your health with *gentle nutrition.*

Additionally, it's important to note that, while many intuitive eating-aligned health providers will agree that intuitive eating can be used in conjunction with chronic diseases such as psoriasis, the undertone is that it's a thin line. It's a thin line between identifying a food sensitivity without recommending a restrictive diet. It's a thin line between suggesting that certain foods may aid in healing without promoting excessive and obsessive healthy eating. It's a thin line to suggest a maximum amount of sugar be followed per day on average while still advocating that you can eat anything and everything you want. I try to tiptoe these lines as cleanly as possible, but if you find any of the sections in this book to trigger feelings of restriction like a diet would, then you should avoid that section and try another one.

Below you will find the 10 principles of intuitive eating paired with a description specific to psoriasis:

1. Reject the Diet Mentality

If you've spent even one minute Googling psoriasis and diet, then you've almost certainly come across a whole plethora of diets that claim to help with psoriasis and other autoimmune disorders. Since autoimmune diseases are chronic health problems, any diet that you can't stick to for a long time ultimately isn't going to heal your psoriasis – and most if not all of the autoimmune diets out there are much too strict to live with forever! Even the "elimination diets" which promise relief from your symptoms after a "reintroduction" period that they claim is easy and straightforward are actually often unsustainable, unhealthy, and unrealistic. While there may be one, rarely two, underlying food sensitivities that are triggering your psoriasis, it is NOT necessary or even helpful to abuse yourself with these wildly restrictive diets. An unsustainable diet will not improve your psoriasis over the long haul – and, in fact, may make it worse by causing you extra stress.[1]

2. Honor Your Hunger

Hunger cues are a critical method of communication from our bodies to our brains. Trying to suppress, change, or otherwise alter our hunger cues will not help heal psoriasis. In fact the opposite is true: following our natural appetite will guide us towards healing foods when needed, and also safe fasting when helpful. Eating regularly plus occasional fasting are both very important to healing psoriasis. These cues must come from the bottom up (from our stomachs to our heads), not from the top down (not from our heads to our stomachs). It's okay to eat less at times, and it's okay to overeat at other times. Both are healing and important. If you have a history of dieting, subtle hunger cues may be difficult to recognize.[1]

3. MAKE PEACE WITH FOOD

While this book discusses many foods that may make your psoriasis feel better or worse, it is not helpful to label some foods as "good" and others as "bad." Instead, what will be most healing is your overall eating pattern. All foods can fit into your life while reducing your psoriasis, and no food should be avoided forever based on some intellectual reasoning like a nutrition fact. As it were, the way to loosen and eventually break the grip that "bad" or "forbidden" foods may have on your psyche is by eating them guilt-free without restraint until you tire of them, without having to "make up" for it later with excessive healthy eating, exercise, fasting, or similar. This may be accompanied by an initial flare-up of psoriasis, but destroying the power that "bad" foods may be holding over you is more important and helpful to healing psoriasis in the long run. Healing your relationship with food is critical to healing your relationship with psoriasis. If you experienced food deprivation of any form in childhood, making peace with food may be more difficult for you.[1]

4. CHALLENGE THE FOOD POLICE

The "food police" can be people in your life and/or the voices inside your head that say you are "good" for eating this certain food, or "bad" for eating this other food. Guilt is often associated with food police interactions. The food police include dieting rules that you "shouldn't" break or "must" follow, a catalogue of extremes that are impossible to uphold every single day. Instead of fostering such a judgemental approach to food and the way we eat, it's more helpful to convert your mindset to making non-judgmental observations and being gentle with yourself. It's about catching yourself thinking nasty thoughts or internalizing nasty comments from others, and trying to redirect that energy into something actually useful and healing. It's about replacing irrational thoughts with rational ones that are centered in learning and curiosity.

Instead of thinking "I shouldn't be eating these cookies even though I really want them because the sugar and gluten will probably flare my psoriasis," allow yourself to think "These cookies are delicious and bring me satisfaction. I chose to enjoy these now instead of stressing over potential health problems; I will find out later if they had an impact on my psoriasis. If so, that's okay – I'm doing better little by little. I can make a different decision about future cookies if I so chose at that time."[1]

5. Discover the Satisfaction Factor

When eating, pleasure and satisfaction should be key ingredients, but they are often neglected and ignored. Eat foods that are satisfying, that you enjoy, and that completely fulfill your cravings. As you tune in more to your body and identify which foods and habits are healing to you, you will begin to crave those foods and habits more because they lower your pain. In this way, you can find enjoyable ways to happily reduce and manage your psoriasis. As you begin to identify exactly how much pain a certain amount of food will cause you (for example, perhaps you can get by with a few bites of gluten without major issues, but know that eating more than that will cause you pain), then YOU can decide in that moment if the enjoyment derived from that food is greater than the joy you will derive from being in less pain later. There is no right or wrong answer – the choice is entirely yours, now and forever! Eat what you feel like eating. This includes, in general, eating before you become starved and stopping before you become uncomfortably full.[1]

6. Feel Your Fullness

When eating, pause and check in with yourself at least once to ask how hungry you still are. You do not need to clean your plate, and instead should aim to eat until you are comfortably full. It may be helpful to explore eating without distractions if it is difficult to determine where your comfortable fullness ends and uncomfortable fullness begins. At times, eating past comfort may paradoxically be enjoyable – like at Thanksgiving – and that's okay, too. Your body will guide you towards more food when it needs more nutrients, and towards less food when its needs are otherwise.[1]

7. Cope with Your Emotions with Kindness

Detangling our emotions from our eating patterns requires that we take a critical look at ourselves. If you find yourself eating when you're not biologically hungry, then try to hone in on the feeling that you're experiencing which is pushing you to eat when not hungry. We might eat to feel comfort, to distract ourselves, as punishment, out of boredom or procrastination, as a reward or bribe, out of excitement, to soothe ourselves, to deal with anger or frustration, when we're stressed or anxious, when we're sad, as a means of escape, for social reasons, or we may eat to prevent ourselves from feeling unwanted feelings. Instead, we are better served if we find other ways to handle our emotions. Regularly engaging in activities that you find relaxing is a great start. Using food to deal with our emotions is a sign that our coping mechanisms are insufficient for the emotion we're experiencing, and it's time we develop new skills to deal with them better.[1] However, that said, it's important to know that some emotional eating is perfectly normal!

Handling our emotions in healthier ways will help reduce psoriasis by ensuring that we aren't undereating, overeating, or eating foods that don't coincide with what our body needs to heal. Instead of masking our body's needs with our emotions, we free ourselves to listen closer to our biological needs which will lead us towards self-healing.

8. Respect Your Body

There's no doubt that living with psoriasis is hard, but we will be better off once we accept our psoriasis and learn to have a less contentious relationship with it. We want to end the mentality that we are at war with our body, and instead trust that it is leaving us clues that lead towards self-healing if we just stop to listen. Since we are constantly bombarded with inaccurate messaging that weight loss will reduce our psoriasis, coming to peace with whatever our natural body size and shape is is a part of this work. Easier said than done when the outside world is filled with fat shaming culture and with people staring at our psoriasis as if we're contagious. We must work towards fostering peace and respect for ourselves – being at war with our bodies won't improve our psoriasis or overall health. Treat yourself with the care, love, and respect that you deserve. Work on speaking kindly towards yourself about your body and your psoriasis. You don't have to be in love with every inch of your body in order to be kind to it and treat it right. This is no easy task, but it is necessary. Joining a support group can be quite helpful.[1]

9. Movement – Feel the Difference

Movement or exercise should feel good and be enjoyable; it should not be a form of self-abuse. If the word "exercise" encourages you to have a firm, regimented, and inflexible idea of what your workout should look like, then forget it and use the word "movement" instead. It's very common for folks who are trying to get back into exercise to overdo it and overexercise, then not exercise again for a while. This is not helpful. Instead, focus on finding ways of moving that are in tune with your body's needs that day. Maybe your body is calling for a round of stretching or a walk instead of an hour sweat-a-thon. Maybe tomorrow you will need something else. Maybe another day you will need a little bit of all of those things. Regardless, any type of movement for any length of time is valuable. Just like eating, ask your body what it needs before engaging in exercise. Focus on what you like about exercising – perhaps improved sleep, reduced stress, better mood, etc. – and find ways to move that help you get more of what you like. Exercise has numerous health benefits, so don't focus on exercising as a way to lose weight. Instead, use exercise as a way to improve your life and health overall. And remember – rest is equally as important as exercising.[1]

10. Honor Your Health with Gentle Nutrition

The best way to truly improve our health is by engaging in healthy habits that we can sustain *over time*. Severely restrictive diets, excessive workout routines, and similar extreme behaviors generally don't (and shouldn't!) last because they're too difficult to keep up with, so we can't depend on them to improve our health over time. Instead, using gentle nutrition and other more even-keeled approaches will guide us towards authentic health and pain reduction.

"Gentle nutrition" means making food choices that are in line with your body's needs in that moment, and eating healthy a majority of the time but not ALL the time. It's about progress, not perfection. It's best to accept that we will never be in perfect health. But, there likely will always be something that we can (gently!) work on to improve our health. Gentle nutrition is a way of saying that stressing over food is more unhealthy than eating something "unhealthy"! Defining food exclusively by its nutrients is simply an inaccurate portrayal of the potential health-giving properties of that food. The key is to eat a wide variety of foods in moderation using bodily cues like hunger and cravings as our guide. The goal is to think neutrally about nutrition, and to make "all food emotional equivalent, even if they're not nutritionally equivalent".[1] The recommendations in the book aim to help you achieve this emotional and nutritional equivalency, even in the face of a chronic disease like psoriasis.

△ △ △ △

Strategy #1: Foods & Nutrients to Eat More Of!

"Let food be thy medicine and medicine be thy food."

— Unknown author
(commonly misattributed to Hippocrates)

△ △ △ △

In the autoimmune world, it seems that we often fall into the same trap, which is to solely focus on foods that we think we should stop consuming. However, it's much more invigorating and helpful to think about *adding* foods! This first strategy is a celebration of the healing power of food. While it's important to reduce foods that are irritating to our system, it's just as important to increase foods that will soothe and optimize our system.

These foods are recommended with the intention of reducing your overall psoriasis and related pain levels. As you explore consuming the below foods and nutrients, check in with your body regularly to analyze if you feel improvement or relief over time. Work on introducing these foods and nutrients into your life more, and once your body is accustomed to eating these foods and has learned for itself what healing benefits these foods have to offer it, then in general you can begin to follow your own cravings and body cues (like flare-ups) to dictate which of these foods and nutrients you should continue consuming and when. If at any point you don't feel a benefit from the food/nutrient, then don't feel obligated to continue consuming it. **You may want to start and stop exploring different sections at different times, based on your perceived bodily needs. You can and should trust your body to lead you in the direction of healing if you're listening close enough.** Use the Calculate Psoriasis Area & Severity Index (PASI) section in the Appendix if you would like an objective way to track the ebbs and flows of your psoriasis.

However, if you have a history of chronic dieting then you may find yourself morphing the following suggestions into another diet. If so, use only what helps you and let go of anything that brings up feelings of guilt or obligation to follow an extreme regimen.

VEGGIES & FRUITS

≫ GENERAL RECOMMENDATIONS ≪

While there is a constant barrage of debate in the nutrition world, the one thing that in general we medical professionals can universally agree on is that fruits and vegetables are an essential portion of any healthful eating pattern. Packed with vitamins, minerals, fiber, and special health-boosting natural chemicals called phytonutrients, you can hardly go wrong by including more veg and fruit into your life. Veg and fruit support long-term health by helping lower levels of inflammation, reduce your risk of heart disease, promote gastrointestinal health, and so much more. Veg and fruits also support your immediate health by giving you more energy, improving mental health, making it easier to wake up, reducing pain in your body, making you feel more clear-headed, and more. While particular disease states may necessitate limiting some categories of fruits and veggies (such as nightshades, discussed in the Strategy #4), there should still be a focus on increasing these health-giving foods.

Actively working to incorporate more veg and fruits into your meals and snacks is an excellent way to set the stage for psoriasis healing. Working to make sure you simply have a veg or fruit present a majority of the time you eat is a great place to begin. Once you are at a place where veg and fruits are regular fare, then you can work to increase the amount. Aiming to fill a third and up to a half of your plate with veg and/or fruit at most meals (but not ALL meals) makes for a good portion.

If you need help learning how to enjoy the taste of veggies and fruits, first I recommend that you find your local farmers' market, especially if it's summer or fall. The best produce can almost always be found at the farmers' market. Generally, the produce at farmers' markets is sourced locally, so it probably only traveled a few hundred miles at most before being sold to you. This allows the farmers to pick the produce when it's fully mature and ripe, which means that the plant had the maximum amount of time possible to pack that little fruit or veg with nutrients and flavor. Foods that travel from far away places are often harvested before they are ripe, so they can ripen off the plant during transport. While that's good for their bottom line, it's bad for our health and our taste buds.

Another tip to help you enjoy veggies more is to season them well! Add salt (yes, salt! It helps with the cooking process), lots of herbs and spices, and don't worry about "cooking out all the nutrients" – some nutrients become more available to our bodies after they've been cooked! If you like your veggies more cooked and less raw (like I do) then don't be afraid to cook them thoroughly. Remember: eating any veggies at all is better than eating none!

Although specific "diets" aren't recommended in this book, it's worth noting that one diet in particular has been studied specifically in regards to psoriasis. This is the Mediterranean diet, which is high in fruits and vegetables and also is not overly restrictive like other diets often are. The Mediterranean diet is characterized by a high intake of fruit and vegetables; plenty of legumes, grains, cereals, fish, seafood, and nuts; low in dairy products, meat, and meat products; and a moderate alcohol intake mainly in the form of wine during meals. Researchers in Italy discovered that "psoriatic patients consumed less [extra virgin olive oil], fruit, fish, and nuts" and "consumed more red meat compared to the control group."[1] This suggests that adopting an eating pattern more akin to the Mediterrean diet may help reduce psoriasis severity. These same Italian researchers also make an interesting case for recommending that psoriasis sufferers increase their consumption of extra virgin olive oil (EVOO) in particular, which has anti-inflammatory properties similar to the pain medication ibuprofen.

While eating more fruits and vegetables may be helpful, it's also important to not become excessive or obsessed about this thought. There will be times when you will eat more fruits and veg, and other times when you will eat less. The average over time is more important than one day. Be honest with yourself, and if you know that you don't consume many fruits and veg on average, then gently challenge yourself to increase the average. If you're not sure, then keep a food journal and write down everything you eat and drink for at least a few days, then assess. If and when you feel that you are consuming a good amount, then your goal becomes to maintain that average. Remember that it's all a balance over the long haul – one day of eating more or less fruit and veg won't make or break you. This mindset allows us to foster intuitive eating principles #8 and #10 – respect your body and honor your health with gentle nutrition – without falling prey to the food police, which is principle #4.

$\cdots$ MORE ON THE SCIENCE $\cdots$

In a 2017 survey of 1206 psoriatic participants, 42.5% of respondents reported an improvement in symptoms by increasing their vegetable intake. 34.6% reported improvement by incorporating fruit into their eating pattern. Additionally, 70% reported that following a vegan diet, which is often higher in fruits and vegetables, conferred improvement on their psoriasis as well.[2]

Improvements in psoriasis due to increased veggie and fruit intake can likely be at least partially explained by their high levels of antioxidants. Antioxidants help to reduce inflammation on the body, and insufficient antioxidant activity has been noted in psoriatic regions.[3,4] Inflammation is heavily associated with psoriasis, and may even be one of the mechanisms behind the fact that psoriasis sufferers are more likely to have cardiovascular health problems and cancer.[5,6,7] What we eat influences the levels of inflammation in our bodies,[8] a concept popularized by terms such as "anti-inflammatory foods." It's important to note that we don't want to vanquish inflammation entirely, as some level of inflammation is absolutely necessary to keep us alive. Inflammation promotes healthy body processes such as wound healing and fighting off infections. However, in general most psoriatic folks would benefit from a reduction in overall bodily inflammation. Antioxidants are one way that veggies and fruits can reduce inflammation in the body.

Another way that veggies and fruits help to improve psoriasis is by modulating our microbiome. Inside our intestines, there is a whole entire microscopic world of bacteria, fungi, protozoa, and viruses that naturally live inside each of us. This colony of microscopic critters is called the *microbiome*. They eat what we eat – so choosing foods that send your microbiome out of balance can also contribute to a worsening of psoriasis. The healthiest microbes – the ones you definitely want living in your intestines – love to feed on fiber, which veggies and fruits are high in. The high fiber content helps support a healthy and diverse microbiome since fiber is food for your microbiome, also called "prebiotics." Our microbiome, which is composed of *trillions* of microbes, is critical in modulating local and systemic immune responses.[9] These little bugs can actually influence which foods we are sensitive to,[10] how healthy our gut is, how our immune system functions, inflammation levels, and even our cardiovascular health.[11] The microbiome's influence is so powerful and remarkable that scientists are actually marking its discovery as significant as finding a whole new organ system.[12,13,14] There is an entire ecosystem of microscopic stuff living inside your intestines – and if that system falls out of balance, that can spell trouble especially for those of us with psoriasis. Eating foods high in fiber helps support this amazing, invisible network of our microscopic companions.

In regards to extra virgin olive oil (EVOO), researchers isolated a specific compound within EVOO that may be of particular benefit to psoriasis sufferers. This compound, known as oleocanthal, is very similar to the pain medication ibuprofen in its anti-inflammatory effects. The researchers speculate that "long term consumption of EVOO containing this compound may contribute to significantly reducing the development and/or the progression of chronic inflammatory diseases and to increase the response to" certain biologic drugs used to treat psoriasis. Additionally, they found that a higher consumption of EVOO was correlated with lower levels of inflammation.[15]

✧ MY PSORIASIS STORY ✧

Although I was eating veggies and fruit regularly when I developed psoriasis, it has still been an important aspect to healing my psoriasis. No other food leaves my body feeling so good after eating it. Veggies and fruit give me lots of energy, they help my mental clarity and focus, and make my body feel great.

I didn't like veggies growing up, but that had to change. I learned how to cook and enjoy veggies by buying lots of them, experimenting with preparation methods, and eating what I cooked. That motivated me to learn how to cook better ASAP! While I don't recommend this strategy to my clients, it is important to learn how to cook veggies so that they are delicious.

Omega-3 Fatty Acids

≫ General Recommendations ≪

An excellent way to reduce the inflammation, redness, thickness, scaling, and overall pain of your psoriasis is by increasing your intake of anti-inflammatory omega-3 fatty acids. Consuming more omega-3s can also improve joint pain, which commonly accompanies psoriasis. In the aforementioned survey of 1204 psoriasis sufferers, 44.6% reported skin improvement after taking omega-3s.[16] Another study demonstrates that psoriatic patients tend to consume higher levels of inflammatory omega-6s and less omega-3s,[17] exacerbating their symptoms.

Foods that are high in omega-3s:
- Mackerel
- Salmon
- Cod liver oil
- Walnuts
- Sardines
- Anchovies
- Caviar
- Flax seeds and flax oil
- Chia seeds
- Hemp seeds and hemp oil
- Oysters
- Soybeans or edamame
- Seaweed

While focusing on consuming more of the above foods regularly may help, my personal experience has been that it's also useful to keep omega-3 supplements on hand, especially during a flare-up. Check out the nutrition facts label to look for an omega-3 supplement that contains both EPA (eicosapentaenoic acid) and DHA (docosahexaenoic acid), as each of these fatty acids provide different health benefits.[18] Look for a short ingredients list, as this demotes the risk that you will negatively react to any other ingredient in the supplement. As for dosing, you might choose to follow the manufacturer's instructions or consider taking up to 4 grams per day during flare-ups. *Please note that omega-3 supplements may interfere with medications like Warfarin or other blood thinners[19] – speak to a dietitian nutritionist or medical doctor about possible interactions with any medications you are currently prescribed and for personalized dosing.*

Top omega-3 supplements:
- Fish oil
- Cod liver oil
- Krill oil
- Algae oil
- Flaxseed oil
- Hemp seed oil

My personal strategy is to focus on consuming high food-based sources of omega-3s often, then take about 1 gram as needed via pill when my psoriasis is throbbing and in pain, and/or when my joints feel swollen and in pain. Always consult a dietitian nutritionist or medical doctor with questions or concerns you may have before beginning a new supplement.

Finally, it's also worth noting that, when it comes to meat, quality matters. Grass-fed beef has been shown to have significantly higher levels of omega-3s than conventionally raised beef. In fact, as grain is increasingly introduced to an otherwise grass-fed cow, the concentration of omega-3s decreases in a linear fashion.[20] Higher quality pastured chickens and their eggs also contain higher levels of omega-3s.[21,22] Although still not considered a top source of omega-3s, if you do consume animal products, then choosing grass- and pasture-fed animal products whenever possible is the best course of action. It's not necessary to consume higher quality animal products every single time you enjoy them, but a majority of the time is helpful. This allows us to follow intuitive eating principle #4, challenge the food police, while still following #10, which is to honor our health with gentle nutrition.

••• MORE ON THE SCIENCE •••

As discussed in the Veggies & Fruits section, autoimmune diseases like psoriasis are associated with increased chronic inflammation. While acute inflammation is a good thing (to help you heal after getting a cut, for example), chronic inflammation is correlated with an increased risk of death.[23] One way to help reduce chronic inflammation is to increase your intake of omega-3 fatty acids, which are naturally anti-inflammatory. Several randomized double-blinded controlled trials found omega-3 supplements improved redness, thickness, and scaling.[24] As discussed in the Veggies and Fruits section, we aren't looking to vanquish inflammation entirely, but instead just reduce it.

Fat is absolutely an essential nutrient – we must consume fat in order to survive. Some types of fat are essential, such as omega-3 fatty acids (also called alpha-linolenic acid) and omega-6 fatty acids (also called linoleic acid). Other types of fats are considered non-essential, as the body can make them itself. Consuming more fat may prove to be beneficial for those with psoriasis, as some researchers theorize that fat malabsorption may be an issue due to imbalances in the microbiome plus chronic systemic inflammation.[25] Personally, there was a lengthy period when I found that consuming a large amount of high-fat foods felt exceptionally healing. However, it is still wise to aim to minimize saturated fats (see Saturated Fat section for more info) and instead emphasize consuming more omega-3 and unsaturated fats. Most plant-based fats are a good source of unsaturated fats, such as nuts, seeds, nut butters like peanut butter, olive oil, and avocado (exceptions include palm oil and coconut oil, which are higher in saturated fat).

Additionally, psoriasis sufferers are more likely to develop heart disease,[26] which omega-3s can help prevent or slow.[27] For those with psoriatic arthritis, research has also shown that omega-3s reduce joint pain and stiffness in rheumatoid arthritis, another autoimmune disease.[28]

✧ MY PSORIASIS STORY ✧

Incorporating more omega-3s – in food and supplement form – has been a total game changer for my psoriasis. Eating more foods rich in omega-3s in general has helped to reduce my overall pain and improve my quality of life. Instead of just sitting there and enduring skin and joint pain especially during a flare-up, taking omega-3 supplements in that moment helps to reduce my suffering fairly rapidly.

Additionally, as mentioned above, it's important to note that a higher fat eating pattern may be indicated for psoriasis sufferers, especially at certain points in the disease process. For me, there was a period of maybe 3 - 6 months where I felt like I could hardly stop eating high fat foods. I stuck mostly to healthier fats – like peanut butter, avocado, coconut, nuts, seeds, and extra virgin oils – but it was like my craving was insatiable. I would just sit and eat peanut butter by the spoonful. Not that there's anything *wrong* with eating peanut butter by the spoonful, it was just out of character for me. In fact, many of my nutrition clients tell me that it scares them when they find themselves eating like this (specifically peanut butter by the spoonful), because we've been told to be scared of peanut butter as it's "high in calories" – entirely ignoring the fact that this is a very healthful and nutritious food! Plus, it turns out that we don't actually absorb all the fat in nuts, so we have overestimated the amount of calories we absorb from nuts by 5 - 30%.[29] Don't be afraid of nuts and seeds – they are so good for you!

However, while on the topic of fat, it's also worth mentioning that during the worst of my *Candida albicans* intestinal infection (more on this in the Sugar section), I found myself sensitive to eating peanuts, peanut butter, and also pistachios. After eating them, my throat would begin to feel congested. It turns out that these nuts in particular can be high in fungi, and since I already had high levels of fungi in my system in the form of *Candida*, I was reacting poorly to the fungi in the peanuts and pistachios. I cut them out of my life for a while, and reintroduced them without problem once my *Candida* was more under control. Visit the *Candida* Screening Form in the Appendix to get a better idea if *Candida* may be an issue for you.

VITAMIN D

≫ GENERAL RECOMMENDATIONS ≪

While vitamin D is primarily known for its impact on bone health, it is also essential for proper immune system functioning. Since psoriasis is an autoimmune condition, low levels can exacerbate psoriasis. However, vitamin D is also not fully understood, and is another hotly debated topic in the medical community. In fact, while we call vitamin D a "vitamin," it actually functions more like a hormone in the body.

At this point in time, the best advice is to request that your primary care doctor check the vitamin D levels in your blood work during your annual physical – and yes, it must be checked *every year*! You can also request vitamin D be checked anytime any doctor takes blood. It may be wise to schedule your annual physicals in the winter, as this is the time of year that levels generally fall to their lowest and supplementing may have the biggest positive impact. Once the results are back, review the labs or ask your doctor to find out what your vitamin D levels are. Most blood work results will mark you as deficient if your vitamin D levels are below 30 nmol/L, but aiming for levels close to 50 - 75 (and less than 125) is now being considered optimal.[30] You may need to ask your doctor what the actual number is in your blood work. If your levels are less than 50, ask your doctor if they will recommend a dosage for a vitamin D supplement. Common recommendations are 1,000 IUs per day or 50,000 IUs per week of vitamin D3 (calcitriol), which is the active form of vitamin D that your body can readily use. Your doctor may prescribe a vitamin D supplement or you can also buy it over-the-counter.

It's best to consume vitamin D supplements with food that contains fat, as vitamin D is fat soluble. For bone health, it's often recommended to take a vitamin D supplement that also includes vitamin K, phosphorus, and/or calcium – whether or not taking these other nutrients with vitamin D are also helpful for autoimmune diseases is unknown at this time.

We can also obtain vitamin D through food – see below for top food sources of vitamin D. The Recommended Dietary Allowances (RDAs) from food sources is 600 IUs per day for everyone ages 1 to 70 years old. After 70, the RDA increases to 800 IUs per day. Our skin can also make its own vitamin D when exposed to ultraviolet B sunlight rays for enough time – but many of us no longer get enough direct sunlight to produce sufficient vitamin D to meet our bodily needs. Plus, factors such as latitude, season, use of sunscreen, clothing, body weight, air quality/pollution, and skin pigmentation affects when and how much vitamin D your skin can actually produce.[31,32] This may help explain why psoriasis is seen increasingly at high latitudes.[33]

Winter may be a vulnerable time for psoriatic folks, as that's when your vitamin D stores are more likely to drop due to lack of sunlight.[34] You may have already noticed that your psoriasis gets better in the summer, and worse in the winter. However, there are some folks who report that sun aggravates their psoriasis – if this is you, monitoring your vitamin D status is even more critical!

Top food sources of vitamin D:
- Wild-caught salmon
- Mushrooms (particularly shiitake and wild mushrooms)
- Eggs (found in the yolk)
- Cod liver oil
- Herring
- Sardines
- Tuna
- Mackerel
- Swordfish
- Beef liver
- Fortified foods (such as: milk, non-dairy milk, cheese, yogurt, breakfast cereals, orange juice)

···MORE ON THE SCIENCE···

Vitamin D helps modulate both the innate and adaptive immune responses, which helps the body to defend itself from harmful organisms and to prevent the immune system from attacking the body, as seen in autoimmune diseases.[31] Vitamin D deficiency is not only associated with increased autoimmunity, but also with an increased susceptibility to infections in general.[31] Since infections are commonly linked with autoimmune diseases,[35] vitamin D helps keep our immune system stronger and more capable of fighting off these infections which may prompt or exacerbate our autoimmune disease.

Research demonstrates that "significant associations between low vitamin D status and psoriasis have been systematically observed".[36,37] One study that was conducted as a double-blind, randomized, and placebo-controlled study found that the group taking a vitamin D supplement had a significantly higher improvement in their psoriasis severity as compared to the control group. No major adverse events were observed, indicating that vitamin D supplementation is a safe way to improve psoriasis severity.[38]

Low vitamin D has been correlated with other autoimmune diseases as well, such as multiple sclerosis, rheumatoid arthritis, diabetes (both types 1 and 2), inflammatory bowel disease (IBS), and lupus.[30,31] Low levels of vitamin D increase the risk of developing autoimmune diseases, and lower levels of vitamin D during pregnancy are linked to increased risk for pancreatic autoimmunity.[31]

Additionally, it may be tempting to try and get enough vitamin D from sunshine alone, but this is a more complex topic than it first appears. The sun's ultraviolet B (UVB) rays are necessary to stimulate vitamin D production. There are increasingly less UVB rays the further away from the equator you live and in the late fall, winter, and early spring. For this reason, if you live south of Atlanta, Georgia then supplementing in the winter months may be indicated. Sunscreen, clothing, air quality, and air pollution impede

UVB rays from getting to your skin even further. Plus, skin pigmentation also impacts vitamin D production – folks with darker skin colors need more sun exposure than a lighter-skinned person to produce the same amount of vitamin D. To attempt to get adequate vitamin D from the sun, you need *full body exposure* for 10 - 20 minutes between 10am and 2p with adequate UVB rays.

Furthermore, even how you bathe may affect the amount of vitamin D that you can make from the sun. Washing excessively with hot water and/or soap can remove too much sebum, which is the main ingredient in your natural skin oil. Healthy sebum must be photoactivated by UVB light in order to produce vitamin D via the skin. If you live close to the equator, but wash off excess amounts of sebum, then you still may be unable to produce adequate vitamin D through your skin alone.[39]

Finally, it may be useful to note that there has been pushback from some providers in the medical community recently, suggesting that the recommended levels of vitamin D (30 nmol/L and above) are too high. While this might possibly be the case for some folks without an autoimmune disease, there is a growing body of research demonstrating increased risk of autoimmunity with low levels of vitamin D. Therefore, for our psoriasis community, maintaining adequate vitamin D levels year-round continues to be an appropriate recommendation. In fact, other medical providers believe that the current recommendation of maintaining equal to or greater than 30 nmol/L is inadequate, and suggest maintaining levels closer to 50 - 75 nmol/L.[30] The topic continues to be debated.

✧ My Psoriasis Story ✧

It's fairly common for my psoriasis to flare up more in the winter, and this is a common complaint of other psoriasis sufferers too. I wasn't sure what to chalk it up to until I came across the above research about vitamin D. I wonder if a major reason why many folks with psoriasis tend to have worse symptoms in the winter is because we're lacking this one little vitamin. I also wonder if low vitamin D levels are a major reason why light therapy can be an effective treatment for psoriasis, as the light therapy stimulates the body to produce more.

Until recently, I thought that eating foods high in vitamin D and getting a good amount of sunlight exposure over the summer would keep my levels high enough. However, over the past few years I have found that my vitamin D levels are still low going into the winter months. Even though I regularly eat foods high in vitamin D (fortified and not) plus intentionally get lots of sun exposure directly on my skin while largely avoiding sunscreen (without getting sunburnt to reduce skin cancer risk) – I have still found my vitamin D levels in the winter to be low. I think one of the main reasons for this is that I live in New York City, and the pollution prevents many of those UVB rays necessary for vitamin D production from making it through the atmosphere and actually hitting my skin.

At my most recent annual physical in December 2020, which I purposely scheduled in the early winter, I again discovered that my vitamin D levels are on the low side. My blood work read 28.8 nmol/L. My doctor recommended 1,000 IUs per day, which I began taking. Once my levels are closer to 50 - 75, then I plan to scale back to 400 - 800 IUs per day, for maintenance. I expect to stop supplementing over the summer months, and begin again in the fall.

As a result, this is a lab value that I expect to monitor for the rest of my life. I have a permanent mental note to request that my levels be measured anytime any doctor does my blood work.

PROBIOTICS

≫ GENERAL RECOMMENDATIONS ≪

Probiotics are a hot topic of discussion so most people have heard of them, but don't actually know what they are. Probiotics are microscopic organisms that, when consumed, are intended to promote the health of our intestinal microbiome. (If you didn't catch it before, the microbiome is the microscopic ecosystem of bacteria, fungi, protozoa, and viruses that healthfully and naturally live on and inside each of us.) While the exact details have yet to be defined, research is beginning to demonstrate that disturbances exist in both the skin microbiome and intestinal microbiome of psoriatic folks.

Does this mean that you should go out and buy a bottle of probiotic pills to help with your psoriasis? Not necessarily. First and foremost, our current scientific understanding of the microbiome, and especially probiotics, is in its infancy. Additionally, there are increasing reports of negative side effects from taking oral probiotics. Instead, I recommend that you focus on increasing your intake of naturally occurring probiotics in the form of fermented foods before trying pill form.

Additionally, it's also critical to feed the beneficial microbes already present and alive inside your intestine tract! The fancy word for microbiome food is "prebiotics," also known as fiber. Our microbiome feeds on fiber – which vegetables, fruits, and whole grains are all high in. Eating plenty of these high-fiber foods regularly will go a long way in supporting a healthy microbiome (find more on this topic in the Fiber section). In general, I recommend trying to include at least one probiotic fermented food into what you eat everyday or most days.

Examples of probiotic fermented foods:
- Yogurt, both dairy and non-dairy versions (Most yogurts will include *Lactobacillus acidophilus* bacteria. Some brands include strains of *Bifidobacterium*. Both strains can be

helpful for psoriasis sufferers – however you should always prioritize avoiding added sugar, particularly found in the flavored yogurts. It is best to stick to unflavored plain yogurt, and lightly sweeten it yourself at home with a natural sweetener like real maple syrup.)

- Kombucha (Again, watch the sugar content)
- Sauerkraut (Buy from the refrigerated section only)
- Kimchi (Buy from the refrigerated section only)
- Miso (Buy from the refrigerated or freezer section only)
- Kefir
- Tempeh
- Natto
- Soft cheeses like mozzarella, gouda, cheddar, and cottage
- There are endless examples of probiotic fermented foods across many different global cuisines – ask about them when you travel abroad! For more information, explore *Wild Fermentation: The Flavor, Nutrition, and Craft of Live-Culture Foods* by Sandor Ellix Katz.

··· MORE ON THE SCIENCE ···

The study of probiotics and their impact on the microbiome is very new and susceptible to drastic changes in the recommended indications, treatment courses, dosing, intake frequency, and so on. It's important to remember that the microbiome is an ecosystem all on its own, just like a coral reef. That means that changing one thing about the ecosystem (like introducing a few fish or a new probiotic) can have various effects throughout the whole system. For example, adding a bunch of fish to a coral reef will affect which plants get eaten more, other fishes' chances of survival, the predators present, and more. Similarly, introducing a new probiotic to your intestinal microbiome affects which nutrients get eaten more, other microbes' chances of survival, which byproducts are in abundance and scarcity, and more. So while research may not correlate one specific microbe to improving psoriasis, introducing that microbe may lead to a cascade of events that supports an improvement in psoriasis symptoms.

The gut microbiome and its relationship to psoriasis is increasingly being studied. While much more research needs to be conducted on this topic, it appears quite clear that the microbes that constitute our microbiome are correlated with psoriasis. At this point in time, the research is as stands: One study demonstrated that the *Bifidobacterium* genus may also be helpful in regulating psoriasis symptoms.[40] There is a case study indicating a relationship between increased *Lactobacillus* intake and psoriasis relief.[41] Another study found decreased levels of the genus *Bacteroides* and increased levels of *Akkermansia* species, *Faecalibacterium* genus, and *Ruminococcus* genus in those with psoriasis, as compared with the control group. This particular microbial disruption may also contribute to a condition colloquially known as "leaky gut".[42]

The microbes living inside our gastrointestinal tract influence many factors of gut health including, but not limited to, leaky gut. Leaky gut – also called "intestinal permeability," a disruption of "tight junctions," or even referred to as intestinal "barrier function" – is one major theory connecting autoimmune disease to intestinal health. Leaky gut is when partially digested food, toxins, or microbes from our intestines passes through our intestinal wall and enters into the body's bloodstream.[43] Our intestinal wall is a very important – yet very delicate – place, since it is only one cell thick. This intestinal wall has the essential function of absorbing water and nutrients for the body by allowing them to pass through the wall. Yet, at the same time, it has to contain all of the microbes that normally live inside your intestines and prevent them from getting in your blood.[44] If the health of this thin intestinal wall is compromised, then partially digested food, microbes, toxins, or other particles can pass directly into the bloodstream. This can provoke an immune response, as our immune system is now forced to work overtime analyzing these particles that are prematurely entering the bloodstream, exacerbating autoimmune diseases. This has been proposed as a possible contributing factor to psoriasis, and there is some research demonstrating that psoriasis and other autoimmune disease sufferers have increased intestinal permeability.[45,46] An overgrowth of the fungus *Candida albicans* can also contribute to the development of leaky gut.[47] Additionally, leaky gut has been noted in non-alcoholic fatty liver disease,[48] for which psoriasis sufferers are at an increased risk.[49] More research is needed in this area. Visit the *Candida* Screening Form in the Appendix to help assess your personal situation.

✧ My Psoriasis Story ✧

Incorporating more probiotics into my eating pattern was one major key to my healing process. To best explain how probiotics helped me, let me describe the background details of my health before I started getting into probiotics.

It was early 2014, and my psoriasis and joint pain were in complete remission just by avoiding gluten. I was doing well – then I took a round of antibiotics for a kidney infection (see the "Introduction to My Psoriasis Journey" in the Introduction for more on this). These antibiotics were the straw that broke the camel's back – my psoriasis flared up like never before, and following a gluten-free eating pattern didn't get rid of it this time. I later learned that, since antibiotics kill off bacteria, they can set the stage to allow a fungal overgrowth to take foothold in the intestinal tract. The antibiotics I had taken in 2011 had likely already weakened my intestinal microbiome and left it susceptible to a fungal infection. The fungus responsible for many fungal infections is called *Candida albicans*. This *Candida* overgrowth further compromised the health of my intestinal tract by promoting "leaky gut,"[47] which made my psoriasis worse (more on leaky gut in the Probiotics section). My chronically stressed life plus habit of eating excessive sugar and gluten led to an intestinal fungal overgrowth, encouraged leaky gut, and took a big toll on my health.

My microbiome had taken a beating, and now I was living with a low grade chronic *Candida* infection. It wasn't until I began to dive deep into learning about *Candida* and treating myself for a

Candida overgrowth that my psoriasis finally began to improve again. I began the hard work of getting my *Candida* levels under control (more on this in the Sugar section). This was the first step towards improving the ecosystem of my intestinal microbiome.

As I worked to get my *Candida* levels under control, I began to increasingly consume fermented probiotic foods. The healthy microbes in these fermented foods help to naturally suppress *Candida* levels, which in turn supports the reversal of leaky gut. Nowadays, I seem to crave yogurt all summer long (I tolerate dairy very well, and enjoy locally sourced plain whole milk yogurt). I also make giant batches of what I call "white girl kimchi," which is my homemade kimchi made with kale instead of the traditional cabbage. I tend to crave this fermented food through the winter months. Kombucha is a staple drink in my household. From time to time I purchase unsweetened kefir (made with either animal's milk or coconut milk), and will enjoy several sips or a small glass occasionally. Miso soup is a favorite during the winter months, and I always keep a container of high-quality miso paste in my freezer. I enjoy sauerkraut occasionally for dinner, sauteed with some locally sourced sausage or kielbasa. These foods have aided my healing process immensely, and I intend to consume them along with new delicious fermented foods I discover over my lifetime.

If you do suspect that a *Candida* infection may be contributing to your autoimmune disease, it is best to be careful with probiotic fermented foods that contain yeast, such as kombucha, kefir, and sourdough breads. Consuming these foods when you're first trying to reduce your *Candida* levels may not be helpful, since your body already has too much yeast. It's best to wait until you have begun reducing your *Candida* levels before introducing more yeast to your intestinal tract. However, once you have begun to get your *Candida* under control, then particularly kombucha and kefir can be wonderful additions to your life. This is because the microbial colonies in both kombucha and kefir are created by symbiotic relationships between bacteria and yeast living in harmony with each other. While I had an active *Candida* infection, it was clear to me that the bacterial and fungal colonies within my intestinal tract were *not* living in harmony with each other or myself – I felt it was important to consume probiotics that do contain ecosystems with happy bacteria and yeast. I feel that adding these foods to my life after I started reducing my *Candida* levels was helpful in healing my microbiome. Explore the *Candida* Screening Form in the Appendix for more information.

FIBER

>> GENERAL RECOMMENDATIONS <<

It may be helpful to increase your intake of fiber to reduce your psoriasis. Fiber supports the health of our intestines and microbiome plus helps to reduce inflammation, all of which can improve psoriasis severity.[2] Incorporating high-fiber foods such as fruits, vegetables, whole grains, beans, peas, nuts, and seeds into daily eating patterns is the best way to increase fiber intake. If you have been eating a low-fiber diet, then it's wise to slowly increase your fiber intake to allow your microbiome time to adjust, which will help avoid short term negative side effects like bloating and gas.

The recommended daily total intake is 25 - 30 grams of fiber a day, while the current average daily fiber intake for adults in the US is only 15 grams per day.[50] Personally I don't keep track of how many grams of fiber I consume each day, but instead just work to incorporate high-fiber foods regularly into most of my meals and snacks. Your bowel movements may be a good indicator of whether or not you are getting enough fiber. You would likely benefit from more fiber if you suffer from constipation, if you find that your stool looks like separate hard lumps, or hard lumps stuck together like a bunch of grapes. These are signs that waste is not moving out of your system fast enough, which fiber can help resolve. Start by eating more fiber from food. If you discover that that isn't enough, then exploring fiber supplements is a good idea.

Top food sources of fiber include:
- Fruits (particularly berries, pears, apples, bananas, and oranges)
- Vegetables (particularly carrots, beets, broccoli, artichokes, brussels sprouts, avocado, sweet potato, potato, cauliflower)
- Beans, lentils, and peas
- Whole grains (such as whole wheat, quinoa, barley, bran flakes, rye, oats and oatmeal, popcorn)
- Nuts and seeds (like almonds, chia seeds, coconut, pistachios, walnuts, sunflower seeds, pumpkin seeds)

If you find that incorporating these foods isn't enough to alleviate constipation or suboptimal stool formation, then a fiber supplement can be helpful, too. Even if you decide to use a fiber supplement, continue to actively incorporate high-fiber foods into your life regularly. The fiber supplement I find most effective and recommend the most often is psyllium husk powder. I suggest avoiding any brands that add colors, flavors, or any kind of sweetener – look to buy brands where psyllium husk is the only ingredient. You may need to go to a health food store to buy psyllium husk. Psyllium husk thickens up when wet, so often the recommended usage is to stir it into a glass of water or another liquid and drink it rather quickly. It's very easy to mix into hot cereal like oats/oatmeal or cold cereal, where the thickened texture is more tolerable and often desired.

A brand name fiber supplement that I also recommend is Benefiber (or a comparable storebrand is a great option, too), which also has just one single ingredient (usually dextrin) without any colors, flavors, or sweeteners. This product does not thicken up like psyllium husk does, and easily dissolves into water, coffee, tea, etc. without making your drink thick. Also, this product is easily found at any pharmacy. Personally I find psyllium husk to be more beneficial for improving my stool formation than Benefiber, but I have clients who have benefited from this product.

Finally, another fiber supplement that I often see recommended by reputable sources is ground flaxseeds (ground is important – whole flax seeds will likely go straight through you!).

··· More on the Science ···

Fiber boasts a great array of health benefits. Fiber helps lower cholesterol and blood sugar, promote regular bowel movements, and lower the risk of colon cancer. Fiber also literally feeds a healthy intestinal microbiome, and a higher fiber intake is correlated with improved intestinal microbiome health. Since intestinal microbiome disturbances are increasingly being correlated with psoriasis,[51] incorporating more fiber may help promote a healthier microbiome that demotes psoriasis production. For more on fiber and the microbiome, see the More on the Science portion of the Veggies and Fruits section.

At least one study has found that those with psoriasis tend to have a lower intake of fiber compared to a control group.[17] It's fascinating to learn that apparently "it is well known that the gut and skin microbiome deeply interact,"[51] so in supporting a healthy intestinal microbiome, you may go on to improve the skin microbiome and reduce psoriasis. A higher fiber intake may also reduce C-reactive protein, which is a marker of acute inflammation.[52]

✧ MY PSORIASIS STORY ✧

Unfortunately for me, constipation seems to run rampant on both sides of my family, and sadly I am no exception. Without going into details you may not care for, I'll say that my digestive system and bowel movement quality seem pretty dependent on my regular usage of psyllium husk. While high fiber foods are a cornerstone of my usual eating pattern, my body seems to like even more fiber than I naturally eat without supplementing. I love to incorporate psyllium husk powder into my oatmeal, cereal, and yogurt on a regular basis. If I don't plan to eat any of those foods in a day, then I will mix ½ - 1 teaspoon of psyllium husk into a glass of water and drink it to keep me regular. While I am not sure if this has had a direct effect on my psoriasis, I definitely feel better when I have regular, well-formed bowel movements.

DIGESTIVE ENZYMES

≫ GENERAL RECOMMENDATIONS ≪

Digestive enzymes are natural chemicals that play a key role in helping break down the food we eat into small nutrients. The digestive tract then absorbs these nutrients so they can go on to nourish our body. Since autoimmune diseases like psoriasis are often associated with suboptimal intestinal health, supporting our natural digestive efforts can be another useful tool in easing psoriasis. Our bodies already naturally make several digestive enzymes that chemically break down the food we eat. By consuming foods that also contain similar enzymes, we promote optimal digestion,[53] and by extension, immune system functioning.

Foods that contain digestive enzymes:

- Pineapple
- Papaya
- Kiwi
- Aloe vera (unsweetened inner leaf juice is recommended)
- Ginger
- Mango
- Honey (However, this is still a source of concentrated sugar and should be eaten in moderation)
- Bananas
- Avocados
- Kefir
- Sauerkraut
- Kimchi
- Miso[53]

While I recommend working with foods first, if you find you need more help or suffer from additional gastrointestinal issues, digestive enzymes are also available in pill form. Discuss with a dietitian nutritionist or medical doctor to determine if a supplement is indicated.

··· MORE ON THE SCIENCE ···

Our mouth, pancreas, liver, gallbladder, and stomach all make various types of digestive enzymes to help us break down our food and extract vital nutrients from it. Our saliva contains an enzyme called amylase, which helps break down carbohydrates and starches. Pepsin is the main digestive enzyme in our stomachs, which helps to break down protein. The pancreas is a digestive enzyme powerhouse, and releases multiple enzymes directly into our small intestine. The pancreas is responsible for producing the enzymes trypsin and chymotrypsin (which help us digest proteins), more amylase for carbs, plus lipase to help break down fats. This chemical breakdown of our food is essential to our digestive system and, ultimately, our survival.

Digestive enzymes can influence the presence of leaky gut[54] and demote inflammation,[55] both of which may be useful for reducing psoriasis.

✧ MY PSORIASIS STORY ✧

The natural enzymes in pineapple were one important key to the puzzle of reducing my psoriasis. Once I had identified that I was dealing with an intestinal *Candida* infection that was making my psoriasis worse, I searched everywhere for answers on how to reduce my *Candida* levels. During an appointment with a primary care physician in November 2015, I explained that I believed I had a *Candida* overgrowth. She educated me on how *Candida* can produce a mucus covering to protect itself from being attacked by my immune system, and even to protect it from being attacked by antifungal medications and herbs! From my training as a dietitian nutritionist, I know that mucus is primarily comprised of protein. I also know that pineapple contains a digestive enzyme that helps break down protein (also known as a protease) called bromelain. Bromelain is the reason why pineapple can taste almost spicy or even be a little painful to eat, as it begins to digest the proteins of the tissues on your tongue. I had a genius idea – I would use pineapple to help break down the mucus membrane surrounding the *Candida*.

I began eating a few pieces of pineapple everyday before breakfast. Especially in the beginning, after eating a few bites I would almost immediately need to clear my throat and often would also have a brief productive cough. Possibly the *Candida* infection was in my throat as well as my intestines. I ate pineapple everyday and immediately felt a sense of relief as my throat opened up more and my congestion began to reduce. I did this for about a year, and over time the throat clearing and congestion became less and less, which was a sign of healing. I truly feel that the digestive enzymes in pineapple were instrumental in the early stages of my healing process. I paired this morning routine with, at first, sage tea and oregano oil drops under the tongue. Please read the Sugar section for more on my *Candida* journey, and visit the *Candida* Screening Form in the Appendix for more on *Candida*-related symptoms.

More recently, I have gotten into unsweetened aloe vera inner leaf juice, which also contains digestive enzymes. This juice was also helpful in my psoriasis journey. For more, please read the Aloe Vera section.

COLLAGEN PROTEIN

≫ GENERAL RECOMMENDATIONS ≪

Collagen is a type of protein that is found in various connective tissues throughout the body, and is the most abundant protein not only in humans, but also across the entire animal kingdom.[56,57] Collagen is found in our muscles, bones, tendons, ligaments, organs, blood vessels, skin, intestinal lining, and other connective tissues.

In those with psoriasis, an increased rate of collagen production has been observed,[57] perhaps suggesting that psoriasis sufferers may have an increased need to consume proteins that can be used to make collagen. Research also demonstrates that some components (called peptides) of collagen help protect and promote intestinal wall functioning.[58,59] To optimize your body's ability to make its own collagen, ensure that you include high-quality sources of protein at each meal.

Foods that contain high-quality proteins:
- Animals products (purchase organic, wild caught, local, pasture-raised, and/or 100% grass-fed when possible):
  - Eggs
  - Fish and seafood
  - Chicken
  - Beef

- o Dairy
- o Pork
- Beans and lentils
- Nuts and seeds
- Tofu and soy products (always purchase organic when possible)
- Pea protein
- Oats
- Some vegetables such as broccoli and Brussels sprouts
- Quinoa
- Bone broth

··· MORE ON THE SCIENCE ···

It's important to note that it's not necessary to consume collagen itself, as the body will create its own collagen when you eat protein-rich foods. However, consuming collagen directly from food is not a bad idea either. This likely explains why bone broth – which is generally rich in collagen – has had quite the field day recently. For vegetarians and especially vegans, it's important to consume a *variety* of protein-rich plant-based foods to ensure that you are regularly consuming all nine essential amino acids, which are components of protein. The average adult needs a minimum of 0.8 grams of protein per kilogram of body weight per day, although your needs may be higher if you are very physically active. You may consider a collagen supplement, however it is likely unnecessary if you are consuming adequate protein as described.

✧ MY PSORIASIS STORY ✧

I'm always interested in learning about the food journeys that other autoimmune folks have gone through, to consider how changes in what they eat relates to their intake of protein and other nutrients, then to speculate how that might impact their psoriasis severity. Some folks report being vegetarian or vegan when their psoriasis initially developed, and other people report that they have seen improvements in their psoriasis by going vegan or vegetarian after their psoriasis initially developed. Personally, I fall into the first group. I was vegetarian for years and vegan for a short stint, and was vegetarian when my psoriasis first became a persistent issue and also when it got worse.

When I was vegetarian, I craved eggs almost everyday. Eggs are actually the gold standard for protein among all foods, as the proteins found in eggs are of the highest biological value. Even though I also regularly consumed tofu, beans, nuts, seeds, and dairy products – my body seemed to be telling me that it preferred eggs as its primary protein source, judging by the intensity and regularity of my cravings. Since I started reintroducing meat back into my life, my cravings for eggs have gone down proportionately. I believe this is directly tied to my protein needs. I'm sure my body was using these egg proteins to synthesize its own collagen, and now uses meat to do the same. As such, ensuring adequate protein intake is an area of concern that I have for those folks who are trying to maintain vegetarianism, or especially veganism, while living with an autoimmune disease, not to mention the possibility of encouraging an eating disorder.

However, I'm thankful for the time I spent as a vegetarian, as that's what prompted me to really learn how to cook, and in particular how to select, prepare, and enjoy many more vegetables and fruits. I continue to feel very appreciative of these skills, even years later. However, over the 2012 - 2013 winter I realized how beneficial following a gluten-free eating pattern was for my healing process, and it became much harder to maintain my vegetarianism. Many vegetarian substitutes contain wheat gluten and my stress levels began to rise as I found it harder and harder to find enough food to eat, especially while eating out or while I was with non-vegetarian friends and family. It became increasingly difficult to maintain this non-essential eating restriction, and ultimately I broke my vegetarianism in order to prioritize eating gluten-free. When I ate gluten, I paid dearly with body aches and pains plus psoriasis. Eating meat does not cause me any pain or negative symptoms. As a result, ultimately it became too great a burden for me to maintain vegetarianism.

While I do feel that returning to eating meat has been helpful for my psoriasis in terms of protein, my personal experience is that these gains are quickly achieved and there's no need to eat a lot of meat. Eating meat (excluding fish) one to three times per week is all that my body tells me it needs. However, I would also recommend eating fish one to three times per week on top of other types of meat, since fish is not only a good source of protein but also is often high in vitamin D and omega-3s (see Vitamin D and Omega-3 Fatty Acids sections for more). When I start eating too much meat (excluding fish), I start feeling sluggish, heavy, bloated, and tired; I try to limit eating meat to a maximum of one time per day.

However, what's been even *more* healing for my psoriasis about dropping the "vegetarian" label has been reducing the *stress* that trying to maintain being vegetarian or vegan placed on me. Let's face it – most Americans love eating animal products, and eat them excessively. American food culture is based in eating animals. It is stressful to try to live your life counter to the mainstream culture. Not to imply that living counterculture isn't a worthy pursuit, but in the interest of self-preservation we must diligently pick our battles. For me, maintaining vegetarianism wasn't a battle I felt I had the energy, strength, stamina, or health to continue pursuing. By introducing more animal products into my life, my stress levels decreased, plus my collagen intake increased. The addition of minimal animal proteins has helped my healing process by increasing my protein intake and by reducing my stress levels.

While I have quelled a lot of ethical qualms I held prior about eating meat in general, it is still extremely important to me to choose higher welfare animal products. You will notice this theme scattered throughout the book. I recommend choosing, whenever possible, animal products that are certified organic, 100% grass-fed, local, wild caught, and/or pasture-raised. There is more on this topic in the Omega-3 Fatty Acids section.

This leaves one question remaining: why does some peoples' psoriasis improve when they *stop* eating meat? For those who going vegetarian or vegan helped their psoriasis, I suspect that they were not eating enough vegetables and fruits while getting too much of other nutrients prior to transitioning to vegan/vegetarian. When they began to follow a vegan/vegetarian eating pattern, they ended up increasing their intake of veggies and fruits, plus possibly also increased their intake of whole grains and fiber, while lowering their saturated fat intake. For all of us suffering from psoriasis, whether you eat animal products or not, there is something to learn here: prioritizing the consumption of protein, veggies, fruits, whole grains, and fiber is critically important and vastly healing no matter what name you give to your eating pattern.

GLUTAMINE AMINO ACID

≫ GENERAL RECOMMENDATIONS ≪

Glutamine is an amino acid, which is a part of protein. Due to a lack of research in this area, at this point in time I recommend obtaining glutamine from food sources. Additionally, the human body can synthesize its own glutamine as long as protein intake is adequate, so if you don't care for the below foods then at least ensure that you are getting adequate protein. Speak to a dietitian nutritionist if you have concerns about your protein intake.

While exactly which foods are high in glutamine is a topic for future research,[60] it appears that the below are promising sources:

- Animals products (purchase organic, wild caught, local, pasture-raised, and/or 100% grass-fed when possible):
  - Bone broth
  - Eggs

- o Fish
- o Beef
- o Dairy products
- o Chicken
- Fruits and veggies:
  - o Corn
  - o Beans
  - o Beets
  - o Cabbage
  - o Spinach
  - o Carrots
  - o Papaya
  - o Brussels sprouts
  - o Celery
  - o Kale
- Tofu
- White rice
- Parsley
- Miso and other fermented foods

••• MORE ON THE SCIENCE •••

Amino acids are the building blocks of protein. Glutamine is the most abundant free amino acid in the body, and is essential for protein synthesis and cellular growth.[61] Since psoriasis is characterized by high rates of cellular growth, this increases the body's demand for glutamine. The proper functioning of immune cells are highly dependent on glutamine as well.[62] Additionally, glutamine is a major nutrient in maintaining intestinal health and reducing leaky gut[63] and also enhances collagen synthesis.[61] In short, psoriasis sufferers will likely benefit from increased glutamine consumption.

✦ MY PSORIASIS STORY ✦

Similar to collagen, I trust my body to make its own glutamine as long as my protein intake is adequate. I eat many of the above foods regularly, including often preparing homemade bone broth. I save bones leftover from other meals in the freezer. I also add other cooking scraps to this frozen mix, like onion skins, carrot peelings, broccoli stems, shrimp tails, and so on. Every once in a while, I fill my crock pot with all these frozen scraps, top it off with water, add a few bay leaves and a good splash of apple cider vinegar, and let it all gently simmer for several hours. After straining out the food scraps, I freeze containers of this bone broth. I pull containers out regularly and leave them in the fridge, using them whenever a recipe calls for broth. I also enjoy making a hot cup of my homemade broth with a good sprinkle of sea salt and a squeeze lemon wedge for a relaxing savory drink.

CHAGA & OTHER MEDICINAL MUSHROOMS

≫ GENERAL RECOMMENDATIONS ≪

At this time, there is insufficient research to make a general recommendation for supplementing with medicinal mushrooms. However, if you are interested in using mushrooms to support your healing process, the best recommendation that can be given at this time is to take chaga tea daily for 9 - 12 weeks, as was studied in the Russian research paper referred to in the below More on the Science section. Please note that there is very limited research on this topic and very little data to support this recommendation. There is much more research that can and should be done on this topic in order to support the psoriasis community appropriately.

If you enjoy consuming mushrooms, it may be a good idea to increase your intake of them. Consuming a variety of mushroom types may be more beneficial as well.

• • • MORE ON THE SCIENCE • • •

Different mushrooms have different properties, including different healing properties. In particular, chaga mushrooms may possibly hold the potential to promote the healing process in psoriatic patients. In a Russian study from 1973, the researchers found that psoriatic patients who consumed chaga mushroom continuously for 9 - 12 weeks experienced a 76% cure rate, plus further improvement in 16% of cases. The authors noted that "chaga is especially successful in cases when psoriasis occurs in combination with chronic inflammatory diseases of the gastrointestinal tract, liver, and biliary system which manifest themselves before or during the course of psoriasis".[64] This research absolutely deserves repeating.

A more recent mouse study from 2005 demonstrates that chaga mushroom water extract significantly decreased levels of proinflammatory cytokine tumor necrosis factor alpha (TNF-α), which is known to be elevated in those with psoriasis. However, this same study also indicates that chaga water extract also increased levels of proinflammatory cytokine interleukin-6,[65] which is known to be elevated in the presence of psoriasis and may prove to be counterproductive to healing.

Another mouse study from 2013 demonstrated that consuming proteoglycan, a compound derived from the *Phellinus linteus* mushroom (also known as black hoof mushroom), also reduced TNF-α,[66] and therefore may be useful in the treatment of autoimmune diseases.

In general, immunosuppressive properties in mushrooms have been observed,[67] which may be of benefit to those of us with overactive immune systems. The psoriasis community and autoimmune community at large deserves much more research on these topics.

✧ MY PSORIASIS STORY ✧

If you are someone who enjoys eating mushrooms, then I'm a tad jealous of you! I have yet to find a mushroom that I really enjoy eating – and will continue to try new ones until I find a favorite! I believe that mushrooms can possess healing properties and that it's important to eat them – even if you don't like them.

We tend to think of mushrooms as plants, but they aren't! They are fungi. Mushrooms are like the "flowers" of the fungi kingdom, as they produce and spread spores that will go on to grow new fungi. If you're a nerd about ecology and biology like I am, then you'll agree that this fact alone makes mushrooms very cool and super fascinating.

If you're already interested in fungi, you might be familiar with a mycologist (fungi scientist) by the name of Paul Stamets. He created a line of mushroom supplements called Host Defense, by Fungi Perfecti. I picked up a bottle of his supplements on a whim before my psoriasis went into remission in the summer of 2019 and tried it out. The blend I bought was called MyCommunity Comprehensive Immune Support, and it includes chaga mushroom. I took a pill a day until it ran out a month later. I didn't notice any significant changes in my psoriasis that I could attribute to taking this supplement. However, it's possible if I had taken a higher dose and/or taken it for longer – like 9 - 12 weeks, as suggested by the aforementioned Russian study – then maybe I would have experienced an improvement.

Regardless, I do purchase chaga mushroom powder and other blends of mushroom powders from time to time and mix it in with my coffee, as they are well known for several different health properties.

ALOE VERA

≫ GENERAL RECOMMENDATIONS ≪

Aloe vera is a highly medicinal plant used across many cultures, countries, and continents. Aloe vera has several desirable qualities – such as being anti-inflammatory, antiseptic, and pain relieving[68] – plus has both topical as well as internal applications for psoriasis. Since psoriasis is often paired with digestive issues,[69] unsweetened aloe vera inner leaf juice can be a simple, yet effective way to improve your intestinal health. It aids in reducing intestinal inflammation, helps to promote a healthy intestinal microbiome, contains natural digestive enzymes (see the Digestive Enzymes section for more), and can also help alleviate constipation.[69] For oral use, the label may say "purified" and/or "decolorized." Follow manufacturer's instructions for use. I'm most familiar with and can highly recommend the brand Lakewood Juices. I often recommend 2 - 4 ounces per day to my clients.

You can also find fresh aloe vera leaf in the produce area of some grocery stores. To use the whole leaf, simply cut it open with a knife and scrape the gel off of the skin. This fresh gel or a commercial aloe vera cream preparation applied topically onto psoriasis can help reduce redness, scaling, itching and inflammation. You may need to apply it several times a day for a month or longer to see improvement.[70] While you can also eat the gel from fresh aloe leaves, please note that it is a strong laxative and even small doses can have negative side effects such as diarrhea and cramping.

While it's common to see aloe vera for sale as houseplants, stick to commercially prepared aloe preparations and/or aloe leaves found for sale in the produce area of the grocery store. Aloe vera houseplant varieties may not be safe to ingest or apply topically. Personally, I tend to use the whole aloe leaf topically and the commercially prepared unsweetened inner leaf juice orally/internally.

• • • MORE ON THE SCIENCE • • •

There is a strong link between psoriasis and inflammatory bowel disease (IBD), including Crohn's disease and ulcerative colitis (UC), which are also autoimmune diseases. Aloe vera may be beneficial in improving outcomes for those with IBD.[71,72]

In research, topically applying aloe vera cream resulted in significant clearing of plaque psoriasis, and furthermore, was not shown to be toxic or have any other negative side effects.[73] In fact, in one study, aloe vera gel was found to be *more* effective than topical steroid creams in treating psoriasis.[74]

✧ MY PSORIASIS STORY ✧

I often recommend unsweetened aloe vera inner leaf juice to my clients. I find it to be gentle, yet effective at promoting healthy bowel movements and digestion while reducing intestinal inflammation. There was a period for a few months when I drank a few ounces of the aforementioned inner leaf juice every morning, and found that it encouraged improved bowel movements. I would also often drink this juice when my psoriasis was painful, aching, and sore, and found that it offered me fairly quick relief.

When my psoriasis would flare up, occasionally I would explore a 12, 24, or 36-hour fast (for more on this topic, please visit the Benefits of Fasting section). During these fasts, I would avoid food but make sure to drink several healing liquids such as this aloe juice. I felt that it amplified the benefits of fasting and expedited intestinal healing.

△ △ △ △

Strategy #2: Meal Timing

"If we could give every individual the right amount of nourishment and exercise, not too little and not too much, we would have found the safest way to health."

— Hippocrates,
ancient physician & father of modern medicine

△ △ △ △

Benefits of Eating Regularly

≫ General Recommendations ≪

We all skip a meal here and there – but meal skipping should not define our regular eating habits. Eating regularly helps support our natural circadian rhythm plus promotes metabolic and cardiovascular health.[1,2,3] Additionally, not eating frequently or eating enough food can be perceived as stress by our body. Our bodies get scared when we don't get enough food – purely as a survival instinct – which promotes the stress response. Since stress is a known trigger for psoriasis,[4,5,6] it's wisest to eat reliably and regularly to remove this stressor from our lives. In general, it's best to keep our bodies at a comfortable level of fullness and hunger at all times. Plan to eat every 3-4 hours.

As a result, I suggest consuming breakfast, lunch, and dinner most days plus healthier snacks as desired to demote the stress response. There are many stressors in life that are extremely difficult to reduce (for example, the loss of a loved one), so eating more regularly is a comparatively easy way to reduce stress! Take advantage of this. To get the full benefit, at times you may need to employ "planned hunger," which is eating even when you're not particularly hungry because you know you won't be able to eat later when you definitely will be hungry. An example of this is if you're going to dinner before a movie and aren't quite hungry for dinner, but know the movie doesn't get out until 10pm and by then you will be very hungry, so you decide to eat dinner beforehand even though you're not hungry yet.

It's important to note that a history of dieting may cause a deterioration of your hunger cues.[7] Focusing on eating regularly will help to support the restoration of regular functioning of hunger cues. In general, focus on eating when you are pleasantly hungry, and try not to wait to eat until you are ravenously hungry. Work towards ending your meal or snack when you are comfortably full and satisfied, not uncomfortably stuffed. If you struggle with emotional eating, then eating regularly and tuning in to your hunger/fullness cues can help to loosen its grip on your psyche – just be sure to replace eating with another safe activity to deal with the triggering emotion. If possible, make sure your fridge and cupboard are stocked with a nice variety of foods for you to enjoy. If you aren't hungry enough to eat all of the food on your plate, then save the leftovers by placing it in a container for later. This supports the intuitive eating principles #1, #2, #5, #6, and #7 which are to reject the diet mentality, honor your hunger, discover the satisfaction factor, feel your fullness, and cope with your emotions with kindness.[7]

• • • MORE ON THE SCIENCE • • •

One of the main benefits of eating regularly is to support proper functioning of our circadian rhythm. The circadian rhythm is a 24-hour biological clock that drives the daily rhythms of our physiology – it influences when we sleep, our hormone levels, and even how we respond to medication. Exposure to daylight plus meal timing influences our circadian rhythm. Maintaining this internal clock is important for long term health.[8] In fact, a disrupted circadian rhythm is associated with an increased incidence of chronic diseases such as type 2 diabetes,[9] and has been found to promote psoriasis-like skin inflammation in mice.[10] Although the reason why is unclear, circadian rhythm abnormalities have been linked to psoriasis in humans as well, such as research demonstrating an increased incidence of psoriasis in night-shift workers and reduced levels of melatonin (a hormone that promotes regular sleep-wake cycles) in psoriasis sufferers.[11] It has also been noted that the hormone insulin, which is released after eating, may be a primary signal in regulating circadian rhythm.[9]

Additionally, eating regularly can promote decreased stress levels. When we don't get enough to eat, particularly carbohydrates, our blood sugar can drop. This can produce symptoms similar to stress like rapid heartbeat, heart palpitations, shaking, nervousness, anxiety, irritability, sweating, and the release of stress hormones like adrenaline.[12] Plus, chowing down regularly supports our circadian rhythm, metabolic health, and cardiovascular health.[1,2,3] Therefore, while fasting may be helpful as outlined in the next section, I recommend practicing it in moderation so that the body does not become overly stressed.[13,14]

At this point in time, the effects of meal timing on the human circadian system are poorly understood from a Western perspective.[13] However, the ancient Ayurvedic system of medicine offers more structure on this topic. In Ayurveda, it is recommended to consume breakfast around 7 - 8am, lunch around 11am - 1pm, and dinner around 6 - 8pm (ideally eating while the sun is still up). However, these recommendations do vary depending on your *dosha*, which can be translated as "the three main psycho-physiological functional principles of the body (vata, pitta, and kapha)".[15] For more information and further explanation, please refer to *The Complete Book of Ayurvedic Home Remedies* by Vasant Lad.

✧ MY PSORIASIS STORY ✧

When psoriasis became a notable problem for me, I was eating too little food in general. While there are also benefits of fasting for psoriasis sufferers, I'm glad I didn't discover this until later. When I first developed psoriasis, I was eating foods that were harming my intestinal health (like too much sugar and gluten), but I also wasn't eating enough food. In addition, I wasn't eating regularly at all. I can place a large part of the blame for this on the erratic schedule that college forced upon my life for promoting these bad habits.

Once I finally graduated and was able to have a more regular schedule again, I began to reinstate a regular meal schedule and soon began to experience the benefits. My mood greatly improved. The more regularly I ate, the less cranky I became. For several years I became "hangry" (a combination of "hungry" and "angry") before eating and was quite irritable when I was hungry, but after eating regularly for some time my body calmed down and this irritability subsided. My family and friends are very thankful that I no longer turn sour when I'm hungry – and I am too! Now, I only begin to notice getting "hangry" if I've skipped too many meals or not eaten enough food recently. It's very apparent that I get stressed out much quicker when I haven't been eating regularly.

BENEFITS OF FASTING

≫ GENERAL RECOMMENDATIONS ≪

Fasting is yet another trend to hit the nutrition world recently. Fasting is defined by abstaining from all or some kinds of food or drink, sometimes for religious or spiritual reasons. Although fasting is a long-held tradition in many cultures and religions, it has still become a trendy topic in today's health spheres. Like most trends, it's supposed benefits have already been overpromised – which ends up obscuring the true *moderate* (but maybe not headline worthy) benefits. For us psoriasis sufferers, it appears there may be some benefits to fasting – in moderation. While short-term fasting may be beneficial, it is not useful and possibly even harmful to take it to the extreme.

How can fasting help with psoriasis? Well, eating is hard on our immune system. When we eat and then digest the food, our immune system has to scan all the food to make sure it's safe and won't harm us. This is a huge job, which is why about 70% of our entire immune system resides in our gut. Therefore, when we are not digesting, we give our immune system a break. Plus, fasting helps reduce inflammation and also helps our body clean out old and dying cells.

While the research is too premature to make a broad recommendation for fasting, personally I often use the 12/12 intermittent fasting format, but *only when my natural appetite allows for it*. The 12/12 format is when you consume all of your food for the day within a 12-hour window, and then fast for the next 12-hour window between dinner and the next day's breakfast. A very easy way to do this is to notice what time you eat dinner, and try to eat breakfast about 12 hours after, as long as your natural appetite allows for it. Don't fret if your eating window lasts longer than 12 hours; the length of the fasting window is more important than the length of the eating window. That's because this fasting period allows for what is known as "bowel rest," or giving our intestines a break from doing work so they can heal and repair themselves. Another fasting format is circadian rhythm fasting, where you consume all your food during daylight hours only. This is easier to follow in the summer, and more difficult in the winter.

I do not recommend fasting everyday – instead, mild fasting at *most* a few days a week is all that is needed. As always, never override hunger cues to force fasting or to push your fasting window for too long. Also, don't restrict your food intake after fasting. It's perfectly normal to find that your appetite increases after fasting and you eat more food than usual. Don't be afraid to eat well or to "overeat" after fasting – after all, it makes sense that if you fast when your appetite is naturally poor, then your appetite will return stronger after fasting. Allow your bodily cues to dictate the fasting schedule and amount of food you consume after fasting – always honor your hunger and go with its flow. Fasting should NEVER be used as self-punishment for being "bad" or any other form of self-abuse. This supports the intuitive eating principles #2, #3, #4, #5, #7, #8 and #10, which are to reject the diet mentality, honor your hunger, make peace with food, challenge the food police, prioritize satisfaction, cope with your emotions with kindness, respect your body, and honor your health with gentle nutrition.

In line with this thinking, when I *found* myself with a naturally poor appetite I have tried a few 24 and 32-hour extended fasts (*always* consuming plenty of water plus other healing fluids rich in vitamins, minerals, and electrolytes like plain salted bone broth with a squeezed lemon wedge, kombucha, plain herbal tea, and unsweetened inner leaf aloe vera juice). I discovered that the 24 and 32-hour fasts were met with a rapid healing of my psoriasis. I have also found fasting to be helpful in healing a psoriasis flare-up due to an acute infection (like after a cough or the flu), of course following my naturally poor appetite at the time. It's very important to listen to your body and only fast when and for how long your body indicates it should be fasting for; there is no need to force it. This again supports the aforementioned intuitive eating principles.

While fasting in moderation promotes gut health and gives our immune system a break, conversely eating regularly helps to manage our stress levels and support our circadian rhythm. Both are helpful strategies, and should be used in conjunction with each other.

··· MORE ON THE SCIENCE ···

The majority of our immune system resides in our gut for good reason: every time we eat or drink something, we are potentially ingesting a pathogen or poison. Until it scopes out the situation for itself, our body has no way of knowing if that fish you just ate has already started to go bad or not, if your salad was or was not teeming with *E. coli*, or if that restaurant you love is diligently practicing food safety techniques or not. Simply put, eating takes a toll on our immune system because it has to make sure we didn't just ingest something that will make us sick.

Research demonstrates that intermittent fasting can decrease inflammation by reducing levels of several pro-inflammatory cytokines related to psoriasis such as interleukin-1, interleukin-6, and tumor necrosis factor alpha (TNF-α), as well as by impacting neutrophil functioning.[16] Recent research has begun connecting the anti-inflammatory benefits of fasting to improved psoriasis and psoriatic arthritis outcomes.[16,17] These particular studies used the Islamic religious practice of keeping Ramadan as their fasting structure: "The fasting in Ramadan consists of intermittent fasting that is observed from sunrise to sunset and is alternated with moments of refeeding. Different from other fasting and dieting regimens, such as caloric restriction, the Ramadan fasting follows the circadian rhythm."[16] "The fasting period is not constant, but can considerably vary from 10 - 11 hours in the winter to 18 - 20 hours in the summer period, with an average of 15 hours... During the month of Ramadan, Muslims consume only two major meals, one shortly before dawn (named Suhoor) and the other immediately after sunset (termed Iftar)".[17] This study found significant improvements in psoriasis severity after Ramadan fasting, and promotes the use of strategies like fasting to treat and manage psoriasis. These researchers used the Psoriasis Area & Severity Index (PASI) to measure the psoriasis improvements - calculate your own PASI score in the Appendix.

Fasting promotes a process called autophagy, where the body gets rid of old and dying cells, damaged cell organelles, and pathogens around the cells.[18] It's like the microscopic equivalent of sweeping, mopping, and dusting. The process of autophagy has been found to be dysfunctional in psoriasis,[19] and so fasting may encourage the body to engage in autophagy in a more regular way.

STRATEGY #2: MEAL TIMING

✧ MY PSORIASIS STORY ✧

I was shocked to see how quick my psoriasis started to heal after fasting. For me, fasting has been the speediest way to get my psoriasis to begin healing – one solid round of extended fasting will heal my psoriasis weeks or even months faster than it otherwise would have healed.

As mentioned above, I have explored fasting for 12, 24, and 36 hours. During these fasts, I ate no food but absolutely had plenty of fluids and electrolytes, such as: unsweetened aloe vera inner leaf juice, kombucha, homemade salted bone broth with a lemon wedge, herbal tea, and of course, water.

I only do an extended fast like this when I find myself with *a naturally poor appetite,* when it's easy to not eat and I actually desire to skip one or more meals (helped by the fact that I have been eating regularly beforehand!). I often discover that I have a naturally low appetite after I have consumed food and/or drink that was damaging to my intestinal health – for example, if it's my birthday and I had a slice of gluten-full, sugar-laden cake plus several alcoholic drinks. I have come to believe that having a low appetite is my body's way of telling me that it needs time to heal, and that eating at that moment will cause more damage than good. Fasting has become an incredibly healing experience.

To give an example of this: I took a trip to Colorado to visit my family in September 2020, while much of Colorado, California, Oregon, and Washington were experiencing record-breaking forest fires. While I was in Colorado, the largest fire in recorded history at the time was raging: the Pine Gulch Fire, which decimated 139,007 acres (sadly, this record was broken in the same summer by the Cameron Peak Fire). During this time, the air quality in Colorado was horrendous. We were constantly checking the air quality ratings every few hours, and only would go outside for an extended period or to exercise in the early mornings when the air quality was better. Inside we constantly ran a HEPA air filter, day and night. (For more on psoriasis and air quality, please visit the Reduce Exposure to Air Pollution section.) During all of this, my psoriasis flared up. I had previously been in remission, and now all of a sudden my belly button, elbows, and ankles burst open with new spots. I was saddened, but not disheartened.

Once I returned home to NYC where the air quality was much better (can you imagine?), suddenly my appetite plummeted. For several weeks, I often found myself desiring to skip breakfast or dinner. I followed this natural appetite, and ate at the meal times that I was hungry for, and other meals I just ate less than I normally would have. Within a few weeks of returning home, this lowered food intake significantly promoted the healing of my psoriasis (for more on returning to remission after a flare-up, see the Conclusion to My Psoriasis Journey section). This was remarkable, because prior to this trip my psoriasis would often improve while I was in Colorado, as my stress levels would significantly decrease while on vacation. However, by this trip I had a better handle on my stress levels, and instead my body was clueing me into a different trigger: air pollution. It seems to me that, as my body was handling the extra toxins that I had inhaled which triggered my psoriasis, my immune system needed a break from working so hard, and therefore, my appetite was lowered. This was the first time I have ever experienced what appears to be a reduced appetite due to poor air quality.

△ △ △ △

Strategy #3: Individual Eating Pattern Recommendations – Food Sensitivities

"If you already have some restrictive thinking about food... an elimination diet is like pouring gasoline on the fire."

— Christy Harrison MPH RD CDN,
Intuitive Eating Coach and Anti-Diet Dietitian

△ △ △ △

How can we determine if a food is triggering or exacerbating our psoriasis? How can we figure out if something we eat on the regular is causing us health problems? Our gastrointestinal tract and immune system are highly complex and sensitive systems. They are so intricate that modern day science still has much more to learn about them, plus how they interact with each other.[1] As a result, there is no one single food allergy or sensitivity test – or even set of tests – that will definitively inform you which foods are triggering a negative response in your body.[2] Certain tests may give us good clues, but unfortunately none are entirely conclusive. Instead, our best tool is our personal experience, which the standard "elimination diet" attempts to use.[2] However, following the standard elimination diet protocol can be dangerous and unhelpful. Luckily, we can use pieces of the standard elimination diet protocol in a watered down fashion to more carefully and intelligently identify a food trigger, if one even exists.

A NOTE ON ELIMINATION DIETS

Elimination diets are intended to help us identify any underlying food sensitivities. Identifying food sensitivities, if they are present, is very important. As you can imagine, consuming foods that you are sensitive to can compromise the health of your intestines. Food sensitivities (including, but not limited to, food allergies) can trigger inflammation[3,4] since they are aggravating to the body. People often attempt to use elimination diets to identify any food sensitivities they may have. The standard elimination diet procedure calls for avoiding consuming several food groups at the same time for a few weeks, then slowly reintroducing them one at a time to identify which food is triggering the symptoms. It sounds nice on paper, but the reality of completing a standard elimination diet procedure is much harder. Let's be frank: attempting to reduce or cut foods out of your life is no fun at all. In fact, it's downright stressful and rather depressing. The purpose of food extends far beyond just nutrition – we use food for enjoyment, to celebrate, in maintaining traditions, with our family, in religious ceremonies, and so much more. Restricting ourselves from certain foods is not easy, and can take a huge emotional toll on us.

During my schooling to become a dietitian nutritionist, my professors absolutely drilled this idea into our heads: food is directly correlated with quality of life. The importance of this concept became abundantly clear during my time working as a dietitian nutritionist in a hospital. The majority of patients in a hospital will get the services they need, be discharged, and go back home. For these patients, we would send them food that should help with their disease state – a low sodium diet for those with high blood pressure, a low saturated fat diet for those with heart disease, and so on. However, some patients never get to go back home because they are too sick. They will die in the hospital. For these dying patients – folks riddled with cancer, ravaged by dementia, left severely debilitated by a stroke, or whatever the case may be – we always make the call to "liberalize their diet." For example, even if they have high blood pressure and shouldn't consume excess salt, we would happily send them a bag of chips if that's what they desired. They weren't going to get any better, so what is the point of abusing them with unnecessary food restrictions right before they died? It wasn't until I stared into the exhausted, hollowed faces of the deathly ill and instinctively cringed at even just the *thought* of restricting their favorite foods that I began to truly appreciate the importance of food to human society. Liberalizing the diets of people who are at the end of their life and allowing them to eat whatever they desire can bring much more joy and happiness into their last days on this earth.

As a result of this training and experience, it has become abundantly clear to me that unnecessary dietary restrictions absolutely negatively affect the enjoyment we derive from life, whether or not you are close to death. Therefore, I do not and cannot advocate for excessive and unwarranted dietary restrictions. Unfortunately many, if not all, of the popular fad diets that advertise themselves as being helpful for autoimmune diseases are extremely restrictive. I firmly believe there is no one-size-fits-all autoimmune diet – instead, each autoimmune sufferer *requires* a personalized way of eating to improve their symptoms. While there are elements to these fad diets that may be helpful, there are other elements that are unnecessarily restrictive. Trying to follow any new diet or dietary restriction is absolutely a stressful experience. To restrict our intake of foods that may not improve our disease state creates even more unnecessary stress – and stress is a well known trigger for autoimmune diseases! You can see how at a certain point an elimination diet becomes counterproductive.

As a result of this, these high stress standard elimination diets are infamously difficult to actually complete. However, they are still a fantastic tool – in fact, the elimination diet method is the gold standard for identifying foods you may be sensitive to.[2] Standard elimination diets require you to completely avoid *all suspected food groups* for about 2 - 4 weeks, then slowly reintroduce each food group individually – a painstaking process. This standard method is exhausting, difficult to follow, hard on your social life, and ultimately stressful – which actually could trigger your psoriasis.[5] Additionally, I have seen from my professional experience that it is so difficult for my clients to slowly reintroduce each group individually, that very often people just give up and start eating normally again before they finish the whole process. They might have found relief from their symptoms during the elimination diet – but often aren't able to figure out which exact food is their actual trigger. What a frustrating and fruitless venture. Plus, the actual process of reintroducing foods can cause anxiety and confusion. Other people find relief from their symptoms but get so scared to reintroduce foods for fear of a flare-up, that they maintain an excessively restrictive diet for too long. **For the vast majority of my clients, and especially those suffering from psoriasis and other autoimmune diseases, I do *not* recommend the standard elimination diet method**.

Furthermore, it's of tantamount importance to also recognize the relationship between autoimmune diseases and eating disorders. There is a definite association between eating disorders and autoimmune diseases,[6] including psoriasis.[7] In one study of nearly 1 million children and adolescents born in Denmark, researchers found that "children with an autoimmune or autoinflammatory disease had a 50% higher [risk] for an eating disorder – 73% higher [risk] for bulimia nervosa, 72% higher [risk] for an eating disorder not otherwise specified (EDNOS), and 36% higher [risk] for anorexia nervosa." The rates were even higher for children with an autoimmune disease that has a gastrointestinal component. This association appears to be bidirectional, where having an autoimmune disease places you at a higher risk for developing an eating disorder, and having an eating disorder places you at a higher risk for developing an autoimmune disease.[7] This same study found that "adolescents with anorexia had a 64%

higher [risk] for autoimmune/inflammatory disease, while those with EDNOS had a 121% higher [risk]." Moreover, these researchers also found that "adolescents with a family history of an autoimmune or autoinflammatory disease were more likely to be diagnosed with an eating disorder."[8] Swedish and Finnish studies found similar results.[6,7]

With such a strong correlation between autoimmune diseases and eating disorders, no medical practitioner should *ever* recommend eliminating food groups unnecessarily to a patient with an autoimmune disease. Even a short period of restricting may trigger an eating disorder, which is an extremely serious medical condition. Eating disorders have one of the highest mortality rates of any mental illness, second only to opioid overdose.[9] Almost 1 person dies every hour as a direct result of an eating disorder.[10] Eating disorders also have a recovery rate of less than half.[11] It is critical that as much care as possible is taken while navigating the delicate balance between identifying food sensitivities and demoting the risk of developing or relapsing eating disorders.

Instead of the standard elimination diet method, my recommendation is to eliminate each suspected food group *one at a time* for 4 weeks, while closely monitoring your symptoms. Notice if your symptoms improve over the course of the elimination period or not. Then, slowly reintroduce the food group you cut out to see if your symptoms worsen or not. This can be a long process (and so is the standard elimination diet), but it's well worth it to better understand your psoriasis triggers. My clinical experience has taught me that unfortunately the foods you consume most often may be the most problematic. As you are reintroducing the potentially triggering food, keep an eye out for other signs and symptoms of maldigestion like gas, bloating, stomach pain or cramps, changes in bowel movements, or other intestinal issues. Other body-wide symptoms to watch out for are rashes or other skin changes, joint pain, headaches or migraines, fatigue, difficulty sleeping, or changes in breathing.[12] If you feel substantial relief from eliminating one food group, it's likely unnecessary to try eliminating a second group. If you *don't* feel substantial relief from eliminating a food group, then reintroduce it to your eating pattern and next work on eliminating a second food group. Just to complicate matters further, it's also important to note that our symptoms may actually worsen before getting better once you've made the appropriate dietary change – yet another reason to work with a dietitian nutritionist experienced in this field.

Keeping a food and symptom journal can be helpful during this time – even if you just write down the last 3 meals/snacks/drinks you consumed prior to a psoriasis flare-up or other above symptom. Later, you can review your notes to see if some common triggers begin to pop up. If you need help, I highly recommend working with a dietitian nutritionist who is experienced in working with unidentified food sensitivities and autoimmune diseases to develop an understanding of which foods are triggers for you.

If and when you identify a food group that triggers your psoriasis, it's critical to understand that this does NOT mean that you can never enjoy that food group again. It's very important to not beat yourself up if for *any* reason you eat any amount of your trigger food. Instead, use it as an opportunity to learn more about your psoriasis and to what extent that food impacts it. As an example, if you find that a gluten-free eating pattern is quite helpful in reducing your psoriasis and then suffer a large painful flare-up after eating gluten, then you will discover exactly how significant maintaining a gluten-free eating pattern is to reducing your psoriasis. If you don't want to experience a flare-up like that again, perhaps you will not choose to consume gluten in that amount again. Or, you may find that the gluten-containing food you ate was delicious and fun and completely worth backtracking for. The choice is completely yours to make at all times, and you can change your mind at any moment. Backtracking may also offer insight into the nuances of your disease process – for example, perhaps you realize that you can have a few bites of gluten every now and then without a big flare-up and decide to enjoy gluten on occasion without huge consequence. **Use backtracking as an extra opportunity to learn what your body does and doesn't need to thrive.** Ask yourself: *how serious was my flare-up after backtracking? How long did it take me to heal or get back to my prior baseline? How much did it affect me physically and psychologically?* You are the expert on your own body, and you can use these experiences to learn more about yourself. This mindset allows us to be more at peace with our food and habits, even when they harm us or cause us pain, and is in line with intuitive eating. It should encourage you to feel that you do not need to be in constant pursuit of health to be worthy. Instead, the emphasis is on minimizing your pain and symptoms enough so that you can live your best life and focus on other things. Our main goal is to reduce your psoriasis over time, knowing that there will definitely be setbacks and backtracking. Give it time. The journey is not linear. It's all a learning experience. This reinforces intuitive eating principles #1, #3, #4, #8, and #10, which are to reject the diet mentality, make peace with food, challenge the food police, respect your body, and honor your body with gentle nutrition.

The below food groups are most associated with psoriasis at this point in time according to my research and professional experience. Yet again this is another area that could use more research.

✧ MY PSORIASIS STORY ✧

One of the hardest and most surprising self-discoveries I made while writing this book was realizing that, as a child, I suffered from a disordered eating pattern akin to the eating disorder anorexia (I am not qualified to diagnose myself or anyone else with an eating disorder, so I cannot say definitively if I had anorexia or not). My disordered eating stemmed not from psychological distress, but from physical distress. I was not at all concerned about my body shape or being "skinny" or "fat," but instead was engulfed in a world where the vast majority of the foods I could choose to eat were packaged, ultra-processed, laden with all kinds of questionable ingredients, had a shelf-life of seemingly eternity, were nutritionally questionable, and didn't taste that good. I had to eat these foods in order to survive because I didn't have much access to fresh, minimally processed, nutritious foods. These ultra-processed foods made me sick. I constantly had a headache or stomach ache growing up. I knew it had something to do with the food, so I would just try to eat as little as possible to avoid the situation.

If you knew me growing up, you would know that I was definitely not eating foods considered to be healthier with any regularity. Instead, foods like breakfast cereals, mini frozen pizza bagels, ramen noodle packets, dehydrated egg drop soup packets, fruit roll-ups, go-gurt, ice cream, and the like was normal fare in my childhood home. Both my parents worked and neither cared much for cooking. My parents did limit our sugar intake, but anything else was free game. School was way worse – I could hardly stomach the reheated pizza oozing with mystery grease, the stale French fries, or the dry-as-cardboard hamburgers – so I opted for either a cookie or an ice cream bar most days throughout all of middle and high school. I remember purposely eating lots of meat because I knew it would probably taste alright and would fill me up quickly. This was my survival strategy. I was plagued with constant headaches and stomachaches which, in hindsight, is not remotely surprising.

My high school boyfriend's mother, Sao, would practically beg me to eat more. She told me that I would feel better and have less stomach aches if I ate more. I considered it, but mostly didn't believe her. Lucky for me, she persisted. Over the next several years, Sao would introduce me to a whole world of food I had no idea I was missing out on. First, as an incredible cook, her home was constantly filled with interesting, new, and wonderful smells that became increasingly enticing. I began, slowly, to try more and more new foods. I was shocked to find that I actually liked some of them. Sao's cooking is largely Vietnamese, Chinese, Laotian, and Mexican – as she is of Chinese descent and a refugee from the Vietnam War – and her husband, Dan, is Mexican. Their kitchen became a hotbed for Southeast Asian and Mexican fusion food. I didn't know it at the time, but I was truly blessed to be in their kitchen, sharing their food with them. Now these have become cherished memories.

Sao got me started on seeing the value of foods, but it wasn't until I turned 18 years old that I decided I *had* to find a way to learn to enjoy more healthful foods, especially vegetables. In classic eating disorder fashion, next I became vegetarian. Vegetarianism and veganism are common stepping stones for those trying to deal with their eating disorder.[13] Regardless, I have come to actually greatly appreciate this time of my life because it's when I learned how to cook and enjoy healthier foods. I cooked all my own food and ate it no matter what – which was pretty good motivation to become a better cook ASAP! I began reading food labels and avoiding strange chemical names. *All* of my headaches and stomach aches disappeared. Thankfully, I never returned to severely restricting my food intake (also known as anorexia) as I had been forced to in my childhood.

My next go around with disordered eating would be orthorexia, which is defined as an unhealthy obsession with "healthy" eating. Now that I discovered the wonders of eating "healthy," after some time it turned into a preoccupation. *That food is not completely "healthy" so I should skip it, right? Yep. Should I ever eat cake again? Probably not. Nothing on the menu at this restaurant is entirely "healthy" so should I wait to eat something else from somewhere else and go hungry for now? Yes, I will.* And so on. I got very lucky again and, while working towards my degree in nutrition, I simply had the realization that this was not okay. Some amount of "unhealthy" foods just had to be allowed, otherwise I felt I would go crazy. So, I let it go. I let less healthy items back into my life. Now, I loosely aim for 70 - 80% of the food I eat to be mostly – but not perfectly – "healthy." The remaining 20 - 30% of what I eat can be "less healthy" – and that mindset IS healthy!

Knowing what I've gone through – and seeing so many of my autoimmune clients experience disordered eating plus unhealthy thoughts and habits around food and eating – is one of the main reasons why I NEVER recommend highly restrictive diets to my clients with psoriasis. It's just too unsafe. When I read something like the list of restrictions in the Autoimmune Protocol (AIP) diet, I actually physically shudder at the thought of removing all of those foods from my life. Again, it's just not mentally safe to do that. While I'm so thankful that so many other people with autoimmune diseases are realizing the power of food to heal and manage our diseases, I strongly feel that attempting to abide by long lists of diet restrictions is absolutely NOT the way to handle this information. We should use something like the AIP diet to guide us in which foods to temporarily stop eating *one at a time* and then *reintroduce before restricting another food* to determine if that first food is truly a problem for us or not.

Eating disorders are a mental illness with a low recovery rate and high death rate.[9,10,11] Even psoriasis is less scary than that. Explore food restrictions one at a time. If you are already restricting several foods, it's time to reintroduce ASAP.

GLUTEN SENSITIVITY

≫ GENERAL RECOMMENDATIONS ≪

Gluten is a protein found in certain grains – specifically wheat, rye, spelt, and barley – that have been associated with a worsening of psoriasis symptoms for some. In a survey of 1206 psoriasis patients, 53.4% reported a significant improvement in their psoriasis after eliminating gluten from their eating pattern.[14]

To test if you are sensitive to gluten, remove all foods that contain wheat, rye, spelt, or barley from your eating pattern for 2 - 4 weeks. Any packaging that states "gluten-free" on the label is a safe bet. If you are uncertain, flip the package over to the back side and search for the allergens listing near the ingredients. Avoid any foods that say "Contains: wheat." Finally, you may also need to read the ingredients list to verify if your food is gluten-free or not. See below for ingredients to avoid purchasing and consuming.

Foods that commonly contain gluten include:
- Pastas (including couscous)
- Breads (including matzo)
- Crackers
- Baked goods (cookies, cakes, muffins, pastries, pancakes, waffles, etc)
- Breaded foods (including many French fries)
- Beer and malt beverages

Also avoid ingredients like:
- Wheat starch
- Wheat bran
- Wheat germ
- Cracked wheat
- Durum
- Farina
- Faro
- Graham flour
- Semolina
- Spelt
- Malt

If an item that usually contains gluten like pasta or bread is marked as "gluten-free," then you can consume that product without worrying about compromising the elimination period. Don't fret if you accidentally have some gluten during your elimination period – just keep going on the best you can, and also use it as an opportunity to learn by noticing if your symptoms worsen or not after the accident.

··· MORE ON THE SCIENCE ···

It appears that some people are sensitive to gluten, while others aren't. For those that are sensitive, the mechanism behind this may be that gluten appears to promote leaky gut in them.[1] (For more background on leaky gut, please visit the Probiotics section.) To better understand how gluten can contribute to leaky gut, we need to learn more about a protein called zonulin. Zonulin helps regulate what is referred to as "tight junctions." Tight junctions are the spaces between the cells that make up our digestive tract wall. The more zonulin we have, the more our tight junctions open, which then makes our intestinal tract more "leaky" and permeable. Gluten is a powerful trigger that stimulates the release of zonulin.[1] In this way, consuming gluten can promote leaky gut, which can then go on to worsen our psoriasis and other autoimmune diseases.

Exactly who is susceptible to a gluten sensitivity may boil down to ancestry. Celiac disease, which is another autoimmune disease characterized by permanent intolerance to gluten, appears to be higher in descendants of Ireland,[15] Sweden,[16] North Africa,[17] Finland,[16,18] and Italy.[19] Although I'm not aware of any research on this topic specifically, if your ancestry hails back to any of these regions, then it might be reasonable to suspect a gluten sensitivity over other types of sensitivities, especially since autoimmune diseases have a genetic component. Even if you test negative for celiac disease, you may still have issues with gluten sensitivity.[20] You might consider asking your doctor to test for anti-gliadin (AGA) and anti-endomysial (AEA) antibodies,[21] however still the gold standard remains an elimination test period.

One popular fad diet for psoriasis is the highly restrictive Paleolithic diet, also known as the Paleo diet. In this diet, you cut out all grains, including those with gluten. Since it's impossible to follow the Paleo diet and still eat gluten – since gluten is only present in grains – it begs the question whether at least some of these folks would gain the same or similar benefits from consuming a less restrictive gluten-free eating pattern instead of the Paleo diet. Again, these topics are ripe for much more research.

✦ MY PSORIASIS STORY ✦

For me, it turns out that one of the largest dietary triggers for my psoriasis is gluten. Removing gluten from my life culminated in a large healing of my psoriasis, plus also a great reduction in joint pain (for more on joint pain, please visit the Probiotics and Omega-3 Fatty Acids sections). Eating gluten also exacerbated the leaky gut that I had resulting from my intestinal *Candida albicans* infection (more on this in the Sugar section).

However, it is fascinating to note that – while I am somewhat sensitive to barley, rye, and spelt – I have the largest negative reaction from eating wheat specifically. If I eat a slice of regular bread made with wheat, I may suffer from a whole host of different symptoms such as increased psoriasis, joint pain, and/or brain fog. However, if I eat the same amount of bread made from spelt or rye, I won't suffer from these symptoms. Yet, if I eat *two* slices of spelt or rye, especially for several days in a row, then I *will* begin to experience symptoms. I can also eat barley in soups without experiencing negative side effects. For whatever reason, I appear to tolerate gluten from rye, spelt, and barley better than from wheat. There are several potential reasons this could be the case, but I won't ruminate on those here.

Although my psoriasis is now in remission, I continue to avoid wheat products while enjoying rye, barley, and spelt products. Soon after I went into remission, I did try eating a slice of pizza on regular wheat crust. Although amazingly my psoriasis didn't flare up, I did experience rather severe brain fog the whole next day. While I may have healed enough where I can occasionally consume wheat, it clearly still negatively affects my system.

NIGHTSHADE SENSITIVITY

≫ GENERAL RECOMMENDATIONS ≪

In the aforementioned survey of 1206 psoriasis patients, 52.1% reported a significant improvement in their psoriasis after eliminating nightshades from their eating pattern.[20] The nightshade family includes foods like potatoes, tomatoes, peppers, eggplant, and spices made from peppers. However, black pepper seasoning and sweet potatoes are *not* nightshades, and can be safely consumed if you are avoiding nightshades.

To test if you are sensitive to nightshades, remove the following foods from your eating pattern for 2 - 4 weeks:

- Potatoes (all varieties – except sweet potatoes which *are* allowed. Watch for and avoid potato starch or potato flour in gluten-free baked goods)
- Tomatoes (including tomato sauces)
- All varieties of peppers (everything from bell to jalapeño)
- Eggplant
- Tobacco (of course not usually ingested, but best to avoid anyway)
- Tomatillos (common in Mexican cuisine, particularly salsa)
- Spices made from peppers (paprika, cayenne, red pepper, chipotle, etc – except black pepper *is* allowed)
- Ashwagandha herb

Don't fret excessively if you accidentally have some nightshades during your elimination period – just keep going on the best you can, and also notice if your symptoms worsen or not after the accident.

· · · MORE ON THE SCIENCE · · ·

The mechanism behind this food sensitivity appears to be a specific chemical that nightshades contain – an alkaloid compound called solanine – which is harmful in large doses. Even though in general the levels of alkaloids in nightshades is low, some theorize that even these low levels may be inflammatory or poorly tolerated by some[22] – particularly if the health of the intestinal tract is already compromised. The alkaloid solanine is a known gastrointestinal irritant, and solanine poisoning is associated with diarrhea, stomach pain, vomiting, and more.[23] It is a well known fact in the food world that solanine levels are higher in potatoes that have a green tint to their skin. This green tint is a food safety issue indicating that the potatoes are older, have been stored improperly, and/or inappropriately exposed to light. Check dark-colored potatoes by scratching off part of the skin and looking for any green patches underneath. Regardless of whether you are sensitive to other nightshades or not, do not eat potatoes that are turning green – instead compost or throw them away, or let them sprout and then plant them in your garden. At this point in time, the evidence in support of nightshade sensitivities is primarily anecdotal and, again, more research needs to be done on this topic.

✧ My Psoriasis Story ✧

Nightshades do not appear to be a trigger for me, and I have never tried avoiding them because I've had so much success with going gluten-free. However, I have had several clients who found relief from their autoimmune conditions by avoiding nightshades. While other healthcare providers do not feel that nightshade sensitivity exists, I absolutely do believe that nightshades can cause problems for some folks.

Dairy Sensitivity

≫ General Recommendations ≪

The dairy food group includes foods such as milk, cheese, yogurt, butter, ice cream, pudding, and more. Dairy is a common food sensitivity for many folks even without autoimmune disease,[24,25] making it even more worth mentioning. In the aforementioned survey of 1206 psoriasis patients, 47.7% reported a significant improvement in their psoriasis after eliminating dairy from their eating pattern and 70% reported improvement while following a vegan diet,[14] which excludes dairy products.

Dairy is used as an ingredient in many recipes, so you will have to ask your waiters and read nutrition labels to ensure you are truly following a dairy-free eating pattern. The easiest thing to do if the food comes in a package is to look at the back side of the package near the list of ingredients, where the allergens are listed. Avoid any foods that say "Contains: dairy" on the package. Additionally, there are often non-dairy substitutes available for many foods that traditionally contain dairy.

To test if you are sensitive to dairy, remove the following foods from your eating pattern for 2 - 4 weeks:
- Milk (including buttermilk, powdered milk, and evaporated milk)
- All cheeses and cheese sauces (such as au gratin and white sauces)
- Butter
- Yogurt
- Ice cream
- Sour cream
- Pudding
- Cream cheese
- Milk chocolate
- Half and half
- Coffee creamer
- Clarified butter or ghee
- Some breakfast bars and protein bars
- Many products with a "cheese" flavoring, like cheesy popcorn
- Some deli meats
- Some breads and cereals
- Some soups
- Some types of kefir
- Donuts
- Mashed potatoes
- Some salad dressings
- Some sherbet
- And more

Don't fret excessively if you accidentally have some dairy during your elimination period – just keep going the best you can, and also notice if your symptoms worsen or not after this occurs.

··· MORE ON THE SCIENCE ···

Dairy is a very common food sensitivity. A majority of humans are lactose intolerant and can't digest a type of sugar found in many dairy products called lactose. It's also not uncommon to have an allergy to the proteins found in dairy. An unidentified dairy intolerance, sensitivity, or allergy could exacerbate autoimmune conditions by increasing inflammation and/or other immune responses in the intestinal tract. Additionally, dairy products can be high in saturated fat, which is associated with a worsening of psoriasis symptoms.[26,27]

However, there is growing research demonstrating that dairy is beneficial to other people's microbiomes by increasing levels of *Lactobacillus* and *Bifidobacterium*.[28,29] It seems that dairy is aggravating to some and beneficial to others.

✧ MY PSORIASIS STORY ✧

Like nightshades, dairy does not appear to be a trigger for my psoriasis, however I commonly see dairy sensitivities in my clients. In fact, I feel best when I include some dairy in my eating pattern – mainly yogurt, half and half for my morning (decaf) coffee, and occasionally cheese. I just may be one of those folks whose intestinal microbiome is happiest with the inclusion of dairy.

A NOTE ON OTHER SENSITIVITIES

The above is by no means an exhaustive list of all potential food sensitivities in those with psoriasis. However, these foods do seem to be the ones that most commonly aggravate psoriasis based on current research and my professional experience at this time. If these don't seem to be upsetting your system, then explore the following.

If you discover that you are sensitive to cereals/grains and certain vegetables (lettuce, spinach, cabbage, some potato varieties, sweet potatoes, carrots, beets, eggplant, and peas[30]), you may be experiencing a cadmium heavy metal toxicity. Folks who experience relief from following a diet that removes grains, like the Paleo or Autoimmune Protocol (AIP) diets, may actually accidentally be treating high cadmium levels. More on this topic can be found in the Reduce Exposure to Air Pollution section, and in the Toxins & Heavy Metal Exposure subsection under the Additional Thoughts section.

If you discover that you are sensitive to simple carbohydrates, nuts, and seeds (particularly pistachios and/or peanuts), then you may have a *Candida* yeast infection present. Simple carbs will feed *Candida*, while nuts and seeds can be higher in mold particles which you can have a reaction to. For more on *Candida*, visit the Sugar section and the *Candida* Screening Form in the Appendix.

If you discover that you are sensitive to many high-fiber foods (whole grains, beans, legumes, whole grains, some vegetables and fruits, etc), then it may be because your intestinal tract is inflamed, damaged, and/or in poor health. Digesting fiber is important, but hard on the intestines, and may be causing you pain if your intestinal health is compromised. Just like the recommendation during flare-ups of irritable bowel syndrome or diverticulitis,[31,32] a period of consuming low-fiber foods may help your intestines heal and reduce inflammation levels. It may be best in the short-term to follow a low-fiber diet until the gut has healed more.

Additionally, an overgrowth of *H. pylori* in the stomach is a subacute infection associated with psoriasis[33] that may cause food sensitivities. Caffeine, spicy foods, and alcohol are all foods that can be irritating to someone with an *H. pylori* overgrowth.[34] *H. pylori* is associated with food allergies in general, too.[35,36] Speak to your primary care doctor, gastroenterologist, or other doctor to get a diagnosis. More on this topic in the Chronic Subacute Infections subsection under the Additional Thoughts section.

Finally, it's important to not forget the possibility of a simple food allergy, which can be diagnosed by an allergist/immunologist. The most common food allergens are milk, eggs, peanuts, tree nuts (like walnuts, almonds, pine nuts, brazil nuts, and pecans), soy, wheat, fish, and shellfish.

△ △ △ △

Strategy #4: Universal Eating Pattern Recommendations – Foods to Reduce

"Healing is a matter of time, but it is sometimes also a matter of opportunity."

— Hippocrates,
ancient physician & father of modern medicine

△ △ △ △

While in general the eating pattern you use to tame your psoriasis should be specifically tailored to you, there are a few universal foods that I suggest all psoriasis sufferers reduce to experience healing. These foods tend to increase inflammation, promote leaky gut, plus demote microbiome diversity and homeostasis. Reducing your intake of the following foods will help promote optimal gut and immune health, ultimately supporting a reduction of psoriasis.

However, it is not necessary to avoid these foods entirely. You never need to say "goodbye" to these foods forever. In fact, attempting to avoid a food forever will paradoxically make us crave it more – don't fall for this trap. Instead, **let *joy* be your guiding light. If consuming a particular food will bring you more *joy* in that moment as compared to the *joy* you will derive from being in less pain by avoiding that food, then by all means *enjoy* that food!** Conversely, if you would most enjoy being in less pain later, then honor your joy by not consuming that particular food in that moment. You can change your mind at any moment about what will bring you the most joy. If you don't know what will bring you the most joy, make your best guess and then pay attention to what happens so you can use that experience as a learning opportunity.

Instead of restricting the below foods based on intellectual reasoning, watch your body and symptoms closely to see how these foods make you feel when you do consume them. To objectively monitor your psoriasis improvements and setbacks, calculate your Psoriasis Area Severity Index (PASI) at various times using the corresponding section in the Appendix. If eating a food reliably causes you pain and flares your symptoms, you may find diminishing enjoyment from eating that food. Allow this process to happen naturally over time. You have unconditional permission to eat any of these foods at any time to increase your joy. You also have unconditional permission to avoid any of these foods at any time to reduce your pain. It may be helpful to note that my experience has been that eating a lot of the below foods all at once (like enjoying the food and drink spread birthday party without restriction) is less likely to trigger a psoriasis flare-up than if I eat a lesser amount of these foods over many days.

If you do choose to consume one of the below foods, you never need to "make up" for it later by forcing excessive healthy eating, exercise, fasting, or similar types of self-abuse. Instead, use food in ways that lets you live your best life. Keep in tune with your hunger cues to guide you at all times. You are the expert on your own body. This is in line with intuitive eating principles #1, #3, #4, #8, and #10, which are to reject the diet mentality, make peace with food, challenge the food police, respect your body, and honor your body with gentle nutrition.

If you have a history of chronic dieting, you may need to seek help from a dietitian nutritionist and/or therapist who specializes in intuitive eating and anti-diet therapies before you can truly maximize the benefits of the following section without falling into the trap of a dieting mentality.

ALCOHOL

≫ GENERAL RECOMMENDATIONS ≪

Research demonstrates that alcohol can worsen psoriasis symptoms, and can contribute to triggering the first episode of psoriasis.[1] Next time you have a drink, take note if your psoriasis becomes painful, inflamed, or gets worse within a few hours or by the next day. This phenomenon seems to be more pronounced in males.

For those who really enjoy their alcohol and can't imagine life without a glass of wine at dinner, I often recommend that they explore natural wine, hard kombucha, or wild fermented hard cider. In my experience these drinks have less sugar and questionable processed ingredients, therefore are better tolerated.

Drinking in moderation is the best course of action. Moderate drinking is often defined as no more than 1-2 drinks a day, but my personal experience is that this is too much to support healing psoriasis. Instead, I recommend a maximum of 1 drink/glass per week or 4 drinks/glasses per month. Drinks with less sugar/sweetness are also less likely to be aggravating.

••• MORE ON THE SCIENCE •••

Alcohol is a well known trigger for psoriasis. The mechanisms behind this may be that alcohol stimulates inflammation, suppresses the immune system,[2] alters the intestinal microbiome, and/or contributes to the aforementioned leaky gut.[3] For more on leaky gut, please visit the Probiotics section.

However, it's possible that natural wine and wild fermented hard cider may be better tolerated by psoriasis sufferers. Natural wine is different from many other varieties of wine. Here in the United States, our government does not require alcohol manufacturers to list the ingredients that they used in their product. Often, regular wine contains added sugar, yeast, preservatives, food dyes, and other questionable ingredients. These ingredients boost the alcohol content, increase the sugar levels, speed up the fermentation process, exacerbate hangovers, and ultimately are simply worse for our health – and the label is useless in navigating these treacherous waters!

Natural wine is different. Unlike conventional wine, natural wine is made with *only* the grapes. In natural wine, the preexisting sugars, bacteria, and yeasts already present in and on the grapes at harvest are *entirely* responsible for the fermentation process. Similar is true of hard cider made with wild fermentation. Seeing as how natural wine and some hard ciders are truer to the natural fermentation process, I view these alcoholic beverages as more in line with other health-giving probiotic foods such as kimchi, sauerkraut, and yogurt. From my experience, hard kombuchas offer similar benefits. However, unfortunately I am unable to find any research illuminating the possible different health impacts of conventional vs. natural wine – so, as usual, we need more research in this area.

✧ MY PSORIASIS STORY ✧

Alcohol is absolutely a trigger for me. It is very common for me to see a flare-up after I drink, sometimes even after just one drink. Sugary drinks are the worst offenders for me, while I best tolerate natural wine and wild fermented cider. I'm thankful that at least here in NYC, it is very common for wine shops to carry natural wine. Plus, a company that sells locally produced wild fermented hard cider – the New York Cider Company – is a vendor at my local farmers' market. I can generally tolerate 1 - 2 glasses of these higher quality alcoholic products 1 - 2 times per month without experiencing a flare-up. I generally just try to avoid other alcoholic drinks.

SUGAR

≫ GENERAL RECOMMENDATIONS ≪

Reducing added sugar is a strategy that can improve our health on multiple fronts. I recommend to all my clients with any autoimmune disease that they work on reducing their sugar intake, especially if they have strong sugar cravings. Research has begun to demonstrate that a high consumption of simple carbohydrates, like sugar, are associated with increasingly worse psoriasis severity.[4] Strong sugar cravings may also be a sign of an intestinal yeast overgrowth (additional info below in the More on the Science section). While I often encourage my clients to follow cravings as they can be healing in many instances, sugar cravings tend to be less trustworthy and more damaging. The goal is to strike a delicate balance of consuming enough sugar to offer long-term satisfaction, while not so much that our psoriasis gets aggravated. This is further complicated by the fact that the more sugar we eat, the less sweet it tastes when we do have it. Therefore, if you find that you consume high levels of sugar, it is best to reduce your intake gradually.

It's important to note that I am NOT recommending excessively limiting carbohydrates here. In fact, **I commonly see people villainize all carbs when what they really just need to focus on is reducing their sugar intake** – I think for many people it's easier to think about restricting potatoes or pasta instead of candy, cake, or ice cream. Severely restricting all carbs is the wrong direction to head in, and is an example of diet culture. This supports the intuitive eating principles #1, #3, #4, #8, and #10, which are to reject the diet mentality, make peace with food, challenge the food police, respect your body, and utilize gentle nutrition.

If you find that you consume high amounts of sugar, I recommend cutting down on your intake slowly. Sugar is quite the substance, as it triggers our brain's reward system and in this way has been compared to highly addictive drugs.[5] To reduce your intake, first identify the main sources of sugar in your life. Consider if there are any triggers that encourage you to ingest that sweet food – perhaps a particular emotion, like stress or sadness or boredom? Is it a habit, like an overly sweet morning cup of coffee? Did you skip one or more meals recently, and now are grabbing something sweet because you're starving and cranky? Take a moment to slow down and pay attention to yourself.

Once you've assessed the situation, we can start establishing gentle nutrition and health goals to begin lowering your sugar intake. Pick one or two goals to slow your sugar intake, and feel free to change them up as needed. Examples of these goals include:

- Save sweeter items for later in the day, so the day doesn't start with sweets.
- When you feel physically hungry, choose a healthier item or meal to eat. Save sweets for dessert, when your hunger has already been satisfied.
- Reach for fruit before sweeter items. You will be surprised how often fruit satisfies your sweet tooth. For the times it does not, then go enjoy the sweeter item you originally had in mind after trying fruit.
- Read the nutrition facts label to know how much sugar is in a food. Look at the "total sugars" and "added sugars" lines to guide your choices. Compare labels of products right in the grocery store to guide yourself towards less sweet options.
- Get enough (or extra!) sleep, so you don't use sugar as a way to try and make up for lost energy.
- Eat at least 3 times a day most days.

- Watch the sugar in drinks. Diluting them is a good option, for example diluting juice with water or soda with seltzer. This can be increased over time after you get used to the diluted flavor.
- Use a measuring spoon for any sweetener that you add yourself, which allows you the option to easily reduce your intake over time. This is great for items like coffee which we might have everyday.
- If a certain emotion accompanies consuming sweets, work to find another way to express that emotion that feels as satisfying.
- As for desserts, consider consuming homemade desserts only. Or, do basically the opposite: consume desserts only when they're free, like at a birthday party.

The American Heart Association recommends no more than 6 - 9 teaspoons (24 - 36 grams) of added sugar per day.[6] However, based on personal experience, for those with psoriasis I recommend in general consuming a maximum of 2.5 teaspoons (10 grams) per day – but still always allowing for times when you will go over! This is a goal to reach slowly and not overnight. It's most helpful to follow these guidelines most of the time, but NOT all of the time. More research is needed in this area.

While it is optimal to keep our sugar intake low, it is not always practical. During birthdays, holidays, celebrations, and other such events, trying to follow a lowsugar regimen can feel like torture and be quite stressful. While sugar is a trigger for autoimmune diseases, so is stress. Therefore, it's important that avoiding sugar doesn't become a big source of stress in itself. So, at times it may be the best course of action to reduce your stress levels by consuming sugary foods while fully enjoying the celebration at hand. It's important to remember that our goal is to consume a low amount of sugar *usually* or *regularly*, but not all the time. Low sugar consumption should become the norm, but we should always allow for exceptions. This supports the intuitive eating principles #1 and #5, which is to reject the diet mentality and to derive satisfaction from your food.

Please note that, as mentioned in The 10 Principles of Intuitive Eating section, this is a prime example of one of the most difficult places to balance rejecting the diet mentality while still fostering healing. It is a thin line and delicate balance of not falling into a diet mentality here. Work with an intuitive eating-aligned dietitian nutritionist if you need support.

···MORE ON THE SCIENCE···

Sugar has a huge impact on psoriasis sufferers. Sugar intake has an enormous effect on our intestinal microbiome, brain function, liver health, mental health, and our likelihood to develop more chronic diseases. Consuming high levels of sugar can demote microbiome diversity,[7] increase markers of chronic inflammation,[8] and promote leaky gut.[9]

One way that sugar can make our microbiome fall out of balance is by feeding an overgrowth or infection (these terms used interchangeably here). The overgrowth of one fungus in particular, known as *Candida albicans* and often colloquially called simply "yeast," can be of particular concern. While some *Candida* is considered a normal part of the microbiome, high levels are increasingly being associated with various health problems. Active infections such as a *Candida* overgrowth can exacerbate psoriasis symptoms and promote flare-ups,[10] and *Candida* is one of the most common intestinal fungal infections.[11] Research has begun to connect higher levels of *Candida* with increased rates of psoriasis.[12,13,14] *Candida* releases certain toxins like candidalysin, gliotoxin, and acetaldehyde which suppress the immune system, are carcinogenic, promote leaky gut, and damage the lining of your intestines.[15,16,17,18] Additionally, gastrointestinal *Candida* overgrowth is associated with elevated levels of the pro-inflammatory cytokine interleukin-17,[19] which is the major cytokine elevated in psoriasis.[20]

What we eat heavily influences *Candida* levels since *Candida* loves to eat simple carbohydrates such as sugar. One symptom of a *Candida* overgrowth is an excessive sweet tooth,[21] so strong and intense sugar cravings can be an indication that the intestinal microbiome is out of balance. A high sugar intake increases the pathogenic properties of *Candida*. When *Candida* senses that high levels of sugar are present, it becomes much harder to fight off. Sugar encourages *Candida* to adhere more to other cells and invade them to extract their nutrients. It supports the creation of biofilms (which are a "'city of microbes' where microorganisms live densely populated and surrounded by an excreted extracellular matrix as protection"), which increases its tolerance to anti-fungal drugs. Sugar also reduces *Candida*'s susceptibility to oxidative stress, which is a problem since one of the main ways that the immune system tries to fight the *Candida* is with attacks of oxidative bursts.[22]

Keeping your sugar intake at bay is one key strategy to preventing and demoting a *Candida* overgrowth. However, it's not just the sugar that we eat. Feeling stress encourages our body to release its own stored sugars – so reducing stress is another key aspect of healing a *Candida* infection. See the Stress Management section for more.

While there are many benefits to bringing our *Candida* levels down to normal ranges, it is important to do so slowly if you are already suffering from an overgrowth. If you find that you consume high levels of sugar, it is best to reduce your intake gradually otherwise you may experience what is colloquially called "*Candida* die-off," known to the medical community as an example of the Jarisch-Herxheimer reaction (Herx Reaction for short). *Candida* die-off is a temporary condition that begins once *Candida* starts to die in mass numbers, which releases a large amount of toxins into the system. Symptoms can include: fever, chills, muscle aches or pain, weakness, rapid heart rate, mild decrease in blood pressure due to vasodilation,[23] itching or burning or pain that temporarily get worse, headaches, skin reactions such as flushing or a rash, anxiety, hyperventilation, low energy, and/or a sore throat.[24] These symptoms can be highly unpleasant, are thought to be hard on the liver as it must now process a huge load of toxins, and it's possible for these symptoms to escalate into a serious allergic reaction. So, it's wisest to reduce your sugar intake slowly instead of all at once to reduce the risk of experiencing *Candida* die-off. Learn more about my personal experience with *Candida* die-off in the next section. Use the *Candida* Screening Form in the Appendix to better understand if you are personally affected by *Candida*.

It's worth noting that there are several highly restrictive fad diets in the autoimmune world that advocate completely avoiding entire food groups that are high in carbohydrates, such as in the Paleo and Autoimmune Protocol (AIP) diets. I often wonder if those who find relief from such extreme diets are really just suffering from a *Candida* overgrowth. Instead of enduring these excessive diet restrictions, they might find just as much healing – but with much less stress – if they simply dealt with the infection at hand. Following a highly restrictive diet in order to treat a *Candida* infection is like bringing the proverbial gun to a knife fight.

It's also worth mentioning that during the worst of my *Candida albicans* intestinal infection, I found myself sensitive to eating peanuts, peanut butter, and also pistachios. These are restricted in the AIP diet. At the time, after eating these nuts my throat would begin to feel congested and swollen. It turns out that these nuts in particular can be high in fungi, and since I already had high levels of fungi in my system in the form of *Candida*, I was reacting poorly to the fungi in the peanuts and pistachios. I cut them out of my eating pattern for a while, and reintroduced them without problem once my *Candida* was more under control. Nuts and seeds are a few of the many foods restricted in the AIP diet. However, instead of subscribing to such a restrictive diet that may trigger an eating disorder, your time may be better spent and your health more improved by investigating if you have a *Candida* overgrowth and treating that directly.

If you identify or suspect a *Candida* infection, coconut oil may be helpful. Coconut oil is naturally high in antifungal caprylic acid, a saturated fatty acid that can help reduce *Candida* levels.[25] However, coconut is also high in saturated fat. While the jury is still out on the health effects of saturated fat, there is concern that it may raise LDL ("bad") cholesterol levels. If you are suffering from a *Candida* infection and high cholesterol simultaneously, it may be wisest to avoid coconut products.

Please know that this is not a complete guide on reducing

Candida levels if you are suffering from an overgrowth, and instead is just an outline of my personal experience. There are entire books dedicated to the topic of *Candida*. I highly recommend that you reference more complete resources and speak to knowledgable healthcare providers for additional information. I recommend steering clear of any advice that would have you follow a highly restrictive diet that is not maintainable long-term.

Beyond *Candida* and the microbiome, there are health concerns that any psoriasis sufferer should be aware of when it comes to consuming too much sugar. First, different types of sugars – such as regular table sugar (sucrose) and high fructose corn syrup – are increasingly being associated with non-alcoholic fatty liver disease,[26] which psoriasis sufferers are already at an increased risk of developing.[27] Second, excessive sugar intake can trigger type 2 diabetes, which is also already more prevalent in psoriatic patients compared to the general population.[28] Third, eating too much sugar negatively affects our brain functioning. It alters our emotional processing which exacerbates anxiety and depression. It impairs neuroplasticity which can reduce our impulse control and drive us to eat more high-fat and/or high-sugar foods. This high sugar intake can create low levels of dopamine which may promote us to overeat in order to increase our dopamine levels.[29] If you suffer from depression or anxiety, sugar can temporarily make you feel better, but in the long run may make your symptoms worse.

Unfortunately, eating less sugar is a notoriously difficult task. Sugar consumption releases the aforementioned dopamine plus opioids into the brain, which are addictive substances. Whether or not sugar is "addictive" like drugs that use similar chemical pathways is up for debate, but regardless, reducing our sugar intake can be extremely helpful in treating psoriasis.

✧ My Psoriasis Story ✧

The first big revelation I had in my psoriasis journey was realizing, after months and months of researching, that I was likely suffering from an overgrowth of the fungus *Candida albicans* in my intestines. The infection was likely in my small intestine, also known as small intestinal fungal overgrowth or SIFO. It took many hours of digging and searching through numerous research articles to better understand the connection between my *Candida* infection, high sugar intake, chronic stress, recent antibiotic use, leaky gut, and worsening psoriasis – and I continue to learn more about this relationship. The importance of identifying *Candida* infections does not seem to be on the radar for much of the psoriasis community, in neither patients nor healthcare providers alike.

During the winter of 2012 - 2013, my *Candida* infection and joint pain were at their worst, and my psoriasis wasn't doing too well either. As described in the Introduction to My Psoriasis Story section, at this time I was getting increasingly ill. Not only did I have psoriasis, but I also had joint pains that at certain times became excruciating. I was losing weight without trying or wanting to. I had recurrent vaginal yeast infections. I have quite the sweet tooth, and during this time it was running wild. I had been working at a coffee shop around this time, which gave me too much easy access to chocolate chip cookies, sweet pastries, plus mocha lattes and other such sweet drinks. My sugar intake was through the roof, and I was intensely feeding my overgrown intestinal *Candida*.

During this same winter, on a whim I decided to try following a gluten-free eating pattern. To my amazement and shock, it *worked*! I went from being chronically ill and about to postpone my last semester of college, to being free of all joint pain and psoriasis while thriving! I was stunned. There was just one little weird thing – and that was the skin on my outer hips. After going gluten-free, my hips flared up with this incredibly itchy rash that wasn't psoriasis. I couldn't stop itching – I itched until I bled. My hips were covered with long red lines from ripping my fingernails into the itchy skin. But – the rest of my body felt so much better. I was like a brand new person, just with absurdly itchy hips. Although I was scared, it seemed that returning to eating gluten was not an option. I persisted with maintaining gluten-free even though my hips were on fire. Later, I learned that what I was experiencing is colloquially known as "*Candida* die-off," an example of the Jarisch-Herxheimer reaction. I'm thankful I stayed the course and continued following a gluten-free meal plan. Soon, my joint pain and psoriasis disappeared – but not for long. I also had yet to deal with my raging sweet tooth, as I was still eating simply too much sugar.

Unfortunately during this time when my *Candida* infection was at its worst, if there even was any objective testing available to confirm my theory that I had excessive *Candida*, then I was unaware of it and didn't have access to it. In November 2015, I did make an appointment with a primary care physician and told her my hypothesis that I (still) had a *Candida* infection – immediately an exasperated and pitiful look shrouded her face. She knew that there was a good chance I was right, and she also knew that *Candida* infections are notoriously difficult to temper. She believed my theory and provided me with several natural treatment suggestions that were helpful – although ultimately it took more than those suggestions alone to finally get my *Candida* under control years later. I'm also thankful that this doctor was able to provide natural alternatives instead of simply prescribing an antifungal medication, as taking an antifungal may have disrupted my already compromised microbiome even more. I now have within normal limits of *Candida*, confirmed by a stool test recommended to me by an integrative gastroenterologist in 2019.

To reduce my *Candida* levels, I had to tackle the problem from multiple angles. I increased my intake of foods that are antifungal and biofilm disruptors, I had to reduce my stress levels, and I had to cut down on sugar. It was not easy. I began my mornings with a cup of sage tea, oregano oil, and pineapple. Sage is useful particularly in the mouth and throat to break up biofilm mucous membranes, like the one *Candida* coats itself in.[30] The oregano oil I took in drops under the tongue followed by small sips of water to wash it down. One of the major components of oregano oil, carvacrol, has demonstrated anti-*Candida* properties.[31] I started with about 2 drops per day and – in the interest of science – will share with you that at first I had terribly smelly farts! However, that's how I knew it was working. Often, when your intestinal microbiome is rapidly shifting as mine was, it will let you know with its smell! Once I tolerated 2 drops per day and no longer smelled so offensively, I began increasing the dosage. The digestive enzymes in the pineapple worked with the sage to break up the mucus membranes biofilm surrounding the *Candida* – please visit the Digestive Enzymes section for more on this topic. I began the arduous journey of eating less sugar. As mentioned in the above More on the Science section, sugar releases feel-good opioids and dopamine in the brain. Retraining your brain to get these chemicals elsewhere (like from exercise, as an example) is no small task.

After several months, when the effectiveness of these strategies began to diminish, I switched up my protocol. I began increasingly taking a supplement called Solaray Yeast Cleanse, which was helpful for several years before its effectiveness wore off. *Candida* is a highly adaptable fungi, and it is common for a strategy that once worked to become less effective as the *Candida* discovers ways to grow regardless. This supplement has some grapefruit seed extract in it, but I began taking a higher dose when recommended by an acupuncturist. Grapefruit seed extract also has anti-*Candida* properties.[32] I continued to pursue consuming less and less sugar. I began adding tea bags of pau d'arco (also known as lapacho) to my morning (decaf) coffee for its antifungal properties,[33] which added a wonderfully vanilla extract-like flavor to my coffee. I worked diligently on reducing my stress levels. Over several years, these strategies reduced my *Candida* to now normal levels.

Ultra Processed Foods

≫ General Recommendations ≪

If you can't prepare it in your own kitchen using minimally processed ingredients, there's a good chance it is an ultra-processed food (UPF). These are foods that have gone through multiple "cooking" processes (extrusion, molding, milling, etc.), contain many added ingredients, and are highly manipulated.[34] They often contain a wide array of questionable ingredients, whose effects on human health have generally been poorly studied. UPFs often include long ingredient lists and additives such as artificial flavors, added sugars, stabilizers, preservatives, and more. Many are ready-to-eat, require very little prep work, and are low cost.[35] Reducing our intake of UPFs will also help us to consume less of ingredients that are undeniably unhealthy, such as high fructose corn syrup and trans fats.

It is best to limit UPFs, but it is not necessary to remove them completely from your eating pattern. If you wonder whether or not a food counts as ultra-processed, flip over the package and read the ingredients. If the ingredients list contains items you generally recognize (such as: corn starch, powdered garlic, salt, etc), then it is likely not an UPF. However, if the ingredient list contains several chemical names (such as: mono- and diglycerides, polysorbate 60, artificial or natural flavors, potassium sorbate, etc), then it is more likely an UPF. Generally, UPFs have longer ingredient lists.

Foods that may be ultra-processed foods include, but are not limited to:
- Soft drinks
- Chips
- Many types of chocolates
- Candy
- Many types of ice cream
- Sweetened breakfast cereals
- Packaged soups

- Chicken nuggets
- Hotdogs
- French fries
- and more[34]

Note that there are exceptions in each of the above categories, and there are other types of UPFs beyond this list. Use your discretion.

⋯ MORE ON THE SCIENCE ⋯

Ultra-processed foods can promote inflammation[36] plus their additives are associated with leaky gut and autoimmune diseases in general.[37] These foods contain little nutritional value, but often are high in calories – they are viewed unfavorably as "calorie-dense" foods instead of the desirable "nutrient-dense" foods.

Research shows that consuming these highly processed products can promote eating faster and overeating.[38] Research also demonstrates an increased risk of mortality in general due to consuming more ultra-processed foods, and also an increased risk of "overall cardiovascular diseases, coronary heart diseases, cerebrovascular diseases, hypertension, metabolic syndrome, overweight and obesity, depression, irritable bowel syndrome, overall cancer, postmenopausal breast cancer, gestational obesity, adolescent asthma and wheezing, and frailty."[39] In short, UPFs are not associated with improved health.

By limiting these foods, you also reduce your intake of questionable ingredients whose health effects we have yet to determine, such as carrageenan. One study on rats and guinea pigs found that carrageenan induced "visible erosions of the entire mucosal surface" and ulcerations, likely due to increased intestinal permeability,[40] which could be a trigger for psoriasis. While we wait for scientists to determine if these ultra-processed ingredients are safe, it's best to consume as little of them as we can.

✧ MY PSORIASIS STORY ✧

Consuming excess ultra-processed foods is clearly not tolerated well in my body. Eating too many of these foods can flare up or exacerbate my psoriasis, and also can promote joint pain. While I do occasionally still enjoy ultra-processed foods (Cheetos, strawberry ice cream, and sour cream and onion chips are my favorites!), I try not to keep them in the house on a regular basis and enjoy them only on special occasions.

One strategy I often use is: if I'm hungry, then it's not the time to eat ultra-processed foods. These foods should not replace a meal. If I feel hunger pangs, then it's time to eat healthier, less processed foods. After I eat something less processed, then I can choose to enjoy UPFs more like a dessert. This way, I can still eat all my favorite foods while maintaining my health. It's a win-win.

Lately I've noticed that, even if an UPF finds its way into my home, it may be a long time before I actually eat it. This is a prime example of intuitive eating. I am not purposely restricting my access to these foods, but instead am naturally limiting them because I know they will irritate my skin and cause me pain. To me, this makes these UPFs literally not taste as good. Achieving this type of mentality and relationship with UPFs is a goal I have for all my clients.

SATURATED FAT

≫ GENERAL RECOMMENDATIONS ≪

The types and amounts of fats that we consume can have a significant impact on our disease process (see the Omega-3 Fatty Acids and Sugar sections for more related information). Research indicates that an eating pattern high in saturated fat can exacerbate psoriasis. You may find that simply reducing your intake of saturated fat to be helpful, while eliminating it completely from your eating pattern is NOT necessary. More research is needed on this topic.

Additionally, while there is quite the debate over the topic, it is generally accepted as fact that reducing saturated fat intake is optimal for heart health. Since psoriasis sufferers face an increased risk of cardiovascular disease,[41,42] limiting saturated fat may be beneficial in this way as well.

Finally, it's important to note that if you suspect a *Candida* infection, the benefits of consuming coconut oil (which naturally contains caprylic acid, a saturated fatty acid with antifungal properties – more on this in the Sugar section) may outweigh any potential negative side effects of consuming saturated fat from coconut, at least until the infection is under control.

Foods high in saturated fat:
- Fatty cuts of beef, pork, and lamb
- Dark chicken meat and chicken skin
- High-fat dairy items (such as whole milk, butter, cheese, sour cream, ice cream, etc.)
- Lard
- Coconut and coconut oil
- Palm oil
- Palm kernel oil
- Cocoa butter

···MORE ON THE SCIENCE···

The mechanism that may make saturated fatty acids problematic is that they promote inflammation and oxidative stress,[43,44] which increases the need for antioxidants. A study done on mice with psoriasis demonstrated when these mice were fed food low in saturated fats, they exhibited reduced psoriatic skin inflammation.[44]

✦ MY PSORIASIS STORY ✦

In my experience, saturated fat doesn't seem to be a significant trigger for my psoriasis, however I do try to keep my intake to a minimum. I often eat full-fat plain yogurt with berries, oats, and other rotating toppings for my breakfast, especially in the summer months. While I do enjoy half and half in my daily decaf coffee, I try to stick to 2% on the occasion that I buy milk.I was raised with whole milk and am used to its rich and creamy flavor, but find that 2% milk is close enough in flavor that I hardly notice the difference. I also try to take care to separate my dairy intake from my coconut intake, just to reduce and space out my sources of saturated fat. I also try to stay away from consuming too many sauces or soups that are cream laden – but still can always make room for the occasional creamy delight! It's about reducing, not entirely avoiding.

When it comes to skin on meat such as chicken skin or pork skin, I also play the moderation game. Since fatty skin is my favorite part of a chicken leg or pork cut (skin is commonly left on in Puerto Rican pork preparations, and my partner is Puerto Rican so we enjoy his cultural foods periodically), I just try to consume these fattier foods on occasion. Personally, I would rather not eat a chicken leg at all than eat a chicken leg without the skin! Finally, I also try to buy the best quality meat that I can, which generally helps to improve the types of fats present in the meat. More on this in the Omega-3 Fatty Acids section.

△ △ △ △

Strategy #5: Lifestyle Considerations

"It is far more important to know what person the disease has than what disease the person has."

— Hippocrates,
ancient physician & father of modern medicine

△ △ △ △

Working to improve the quality of the food we eat without also working on our lifestyle is like growing a garden but never fertilizing it. While changing what we eat can be an incredibly healing process, there is more work that can and should be done to holistically address psoriasis. Honestly assessing our mental health is essential. Below I address stress, as this is a huge risk factor and trigger for psoriasis. However, please seek a licensed therapist if and when you need support dealing with emotional concerns. Working on other aspects of your physical and mental health beyond food is another key part of healing from psoriasis.

STRESS MANAGEMENT

» GENERAL RECOMMENDATIONS «

Stress – and in particular dealing with stress – are tricky topics. Stress is not directly measurable. It's subjective, not objective. As a result, many healthcare providers tend to ignore the extreme negative health impacts of stress because it's so difficult to assess and because they often have very limited time with each patient. Plus, we all respond to stressors differently, so one person may handle a stressful event well while another person handles that same stressful event poorly. Ultimately, only you can determine what your true stress levels are.

There are so many different tools we can use to manage our stress levels. Exercise is a great example of such a tool, and is explored in full in the Intuitive Exercise section. An eating pattern replete with healing foods and nutrients is another strategy to help our bodies handle stress better – see the Strategy #1 for related info. Don't forget about the power of eating regularly a majority of the time to reduce stress – see Strategy #2. Meditation is an extremely powerful antidote to stress – see the next section on Meditation. Dieting has been correlated with increased levels of stress and social anxiety, and should be avoided entirely.[1] Limiting your caffeine intake may help, as well as making sure you get enough sleep[2] – see the Get Plenty of Sleep section for more. Other stress-reducing activities worth exploring include journaling, creative outlets like painting or making music, and aiming to laugh more. Forest bathing, or Shinrin-yoku in Japanese, is a popular stress reducing technique that is supported by research.[3] Seeking professional help from a therapist is another great option.

Within the dietary world, an important mineral to consider when discussing stress is magnesium. Magnesium has stress-reducing properties[4] and is considered a common deficiency in Westernized societies.[5] Work on increasing your intake of foods high in magnesium, like:

- Chocolate (I recommend dark chocolate for the lower sugar content and/or unsweetened cacao nibs)
- Nuts (such as cashews, Brazil nuts, and almonds)
- Seeds (such as flax, pumpkin, and chia seeds)
- Tofu (ideally organic)
- Banana
- Avocado
- Leafy greens (such as kale, spinach, collard greens, turnip greens, mustard greens)
- Legumes (such as lentils, beans, chickpeas, peas and soybeans)
- Whole grains (such as whole wheat, oats, barley, buckwheat, quinoa)
- Fatty fish (such as salmon, mackerel, halibut)

Magnesium supplements are also available.

Other supplements that can be helpful in managing stress are CBD and adaptogens. CBD, or cannabidiol, actually contains immunosuppressive properties. This is helpful in psoriasis, where the immune system is overactive. I also often steer my clients towards adaptogen herbs. These are herbs that help the body handle stress.[6,7] I regularly recommend ashwagandha – which has been shown to significantly reduce stress levels[8] – as it is affordable and easily purchased in pill or tincture form. Ashwagandha is prized for its ability to improve wakefulness during the day, but also promotes restful sleep at night. However, if you find that you are sensitive to nightshades, then it's best to avoid ashwagandha as it is a nightshade.

Beyond ashwagandha, another great adaptogen is reishi mushroom, which is known for its immune-stimulating properties.[9] I like mixing adaptogenic mushroom powders into my morning coffee. Other examples of adaptogens include turmeric, holy basil/tulsi, ginseng, astragalus, cordyceps, goji berries, licorice root, and more. For those who suffer from psoriatic arthritis, adaptogens have been shown by research to effectively reduce inflammation and pain associated with arthritis.[7]

··· MORE ON THE SCIENCE ···

Learning to accurately understand and actively reduce our stress levels is an essential component of long-term healing and disease management. In fact, many people with psoriasis report that the disease first became a problem for them during a particularly stressful time in their life, with one study finding that almost half of the patients first experienced psoriasis during a stressful period.[10] Researchers recommend that stress reduction should be a component of psoriasis treatment.[11] Stress appears to cause a delayed worsening of symptoms, where your psoriasis may flare up 4 weeks after the initial stressor.[12]

CBD should be of particular interest to those with autoimmune diseases, since it not only helps reduce stress, but also actually helps suppress our overactive immune systems.[13,14] CBD has been shown to suppress T cell function,[14] where excessive T cell activity is one of the underlying mechanisms of psoriasis.[15] It has also been shown to help reduce the production of psoriasis on the skin level.[16] CBD is being used increasingly to help manage stress, and has been shown to help in anxiety disorders.[13] In these ways, CBD oil used both orally and topically may be of particular benefit to those suffering from psoriasis.

It is of note that research consistently demonstrates the calming effect of exercise, which can last several hours after a 20 - 30 minute session of aerobic exercise.[17] A meta-analysis of over 200 studies found that utilizing mediation was "especially effective" in reducing stress, depression, and anxiety.[18] If you are interested in a more tangible way to assess your stress levels, you could consider asking your doctor to order a test for C-reactive protein (CRP). This is a measure of inflammation in the body, and elevated levels have been associated with psychological distress and depression.[19]

✧ My Psoriasis Story ✧

Stress management has been, and continues to be, a huge trigger for me. Stress was a major contributor to my initial development of psoriasis, and also to innumerable subsequent flare-ups. Anxiety seems to run in my family, so I was raised in an environment that promoted anxious ways of being and living. Additionally, the culture of the United States is deeply steeped in ideologies that promote stressful living in many forms, such as workaholism, valuing being "busy," devaluing slowing down and relaxing, viewing "doing nothing" as a "waste of time," and a "work hard, play hard" mindset. These environmental factors played a large role in the way that I interacted with my world as a teenager and young adult, and I pushed myself to work hard... too hard, I would come to find out.

Since a stressed out mindset was so ingrained into my psyche at such a young age, at first it was extremely difficult for me to tease out first *when* I was feeling stressed, and then to develop coping mechanisms. Of course I still get stressed out, but now I know 1) how to identify when I am stressed and 2) what my options are for doing something about it.

There have been a few key moments in my life that helped me learn a great deal about my own stress levels. I distinctly recall one time I returned back home to NYC from a much needed vacation in the beautiful Grand Canyon. While I was an anxious wreck during the trip, and honestly rather a terror to my poor trip companions, apparently I did relax a significant amount by the end of the trip. It was, after all, truly a spiritual experience – the Grand Canyon is awe-inspiring, magnificent, and humbling. I had planned my itinerary so that I returned home on a Sunday, and went straight to work Monday morning (another thing I never do anymore – now I always give myself a full day between returning home and going back to work!). On my commute that Monday morning, I couldn't bring myself to race to catch my train like I used to. Instead, I slowed down. I noticed the sights, the sounds, the smells for seemingly the first time. It's like I was a whole new person in the same old body, on my same old but somehow new commute to work. It was at that moment I realized how stressed I had let myself become. What's the worst that could happen if I was late to work? Well, I would just stay late. Not so bad. Why was I rushing around as if my life depended on it? I had to change.

My next job was working in a hospital. It was a community hospital in a low-income neighborhood that was clearly on the precipice of physical and financial collapse. As a result, there were few resources among the understaffed employees who were taking care of many sick people. This was an incredibly stressful work environment. It was literally life and death situations all day long, working at 110% of my energy levels every day. I started to develop stress headaches for the first time in my life. My psoriasis was raging. I was, again, overworked and under-rested. The stress headaches were my biggest clue that I simply could not continue working like this. Eventually, I had the opportunity to quit.

While I was quitting, I had the wonderful fortune of already being enrolled in a yoga teacher training at Jaya Yoga Center in Brooklyn. The training was around 5 months long, and I quit my job about half way through the training. Not only did my stress levels drop immediately once I quit working, but the next few months after were followed with a deep practice of yoga poses, various types of meditations, many yoga classes, and the study of yogic philosophy. By the end of my yoga teacher training, a patch of psoriasis that had been on my right ankle for several years simply disappeared. My understanding of stress and its effect on my psoriasis grew exponentially during this time.

MEDITATION

≫ GENERAL RECOMMENDATIONS ≪

Meditation is the practice of and a technique for focusing yet resting the mind, observing the world without judgement, and maintaining a one-pointed focus so that the mind becomes silent in order to increase an overall awareness. Meditation is a beautiful life-long practice that serves to improve our mental health, and by extension, improve our physical health. Meditation gives us a space to assess our reactions, emotions, and habits without judgement or criticism – instead, it just encourages us to simply notice, pay attention, and observe ourselves. Traditionally, focusing on the breath – paying attention to our inhales, our exhales, the way they float our belly up and down, the sensations in the nose as the air moves, the minute changes in these sensations over time, and so on – is a common focal point for meditation. However, there are innumerable ways to meditate.

For the psoriasis sufferer, meditation is one way that we can better understand our stress levels. Through meditation, we learn more about our relationship with stress by developing stronger powers of observation, especially self-observation. Meditation helps us to begin to understand *when* we're stressed, what that *feels* like in our body, and also how we feel when we're *not* stressed. Meditation gives us tools to better understand how stress is present in our lives, and how it is impacting us.

Meditation can also help us come to terms with the profound pain that psoriasis has caused us. As you well know, psoriasis can be a deeply painful condition, both physically and psychologically. Whether you're battling a constant itch, persistent aching and bleeding, depression, or feeling embarrassed and scared to leave the house, there is no doubt that life with psoriasis is hard. Living with this chronic pain can desensitize us to our own symptoms, as we try to ignore the pain signals so we can just get on with other parts of our lives. Ignoring our symptoms can make them easier to tolerate. Unfortunately, this survival technique may also make us disassociate from our bodies. It can turn listening to our symptoms into an emotional trigger, perhaps by feeling betrayed by our own bodies.[20] Meditation can provide us with tools to handle this heavy psychological load. With its emphasis on observation without judgement, we may eventually find the space to approach our bodies again.

While acknowledging our symptoms can be difficult, upsetting, and painful, it can also lend us insight into healing. After all, a flare-up is just a sign that we did something to our body that it didn't like, and if we can start to see a pattern behind our flare-ups, then we can use our flare-ups to identify our triggers. Once we have identified our triggers, then that gives us the opportunity to reduce our flare-ups and ultimately our overall pain. Meditation can help facilitate this process, moving us from ignoring the body towards learning to identify our triggers from our flare-ups. Then, we can harness this knowledge we've gained about our body to reduce exposure to our triggers.

Practicing meditation is difficult, and there are so many ways to do it. If you're new to meditation, then I recommend first exploring guided meditations, where you will be talked to and directed through the experience. There are several guided meditation apps available today. Breathing exercises and breath control are also excellent types of meditation to practice. In the world of yoga, practitioners are encouraged to work with the breath (called Prāṇāyāma in Sanskrit). Deep breathing and slow exhales send relaxation messages to your body,[21,22] both of which are facets of Prāṇāyāma. Square breathing, or Sama Vritti in Sanskrit, is a great place to start. There are many resources online to further guide you in these techniques. For guided meditations on eating, please visit my website at www.autoimmuneeats.com.

If you need help getting into meditation, I recommend completing a 40-day sādhanā that incorporates meditation. "Sādhanā" means practice. In your 40-day sādhanā, push yourself to find some time to meditate every day for 40 days straight. Even 30 seconds of meditating counts. By challenging yourself to try something for 40 days in a row, you are forced to deal with and move through any inertia you may be feeling, and break through to the other side. Then you can more accurately assess if meditation actually benefited your life over those 40 days, and with that information you can decide if you would like to continue with your practice in any way.

It takes time to develop the skills that meditation is trying to teach us, but it is an incredible tool that is worth spending a lifetime practicing. Don't give up if you get discouraged at first. At the beginning, you will likely feel like you can't do it, as you find yourself becoming distracted away from your primary focus within a matter of seconds. Even still, time spent trying to meditate is *never* time wasted.

• • • MORE ON THE SCIENCE • • •

Not only does meditation stand the test of time, as it has been practiced for thousands of years, but modern-day science and research only further confirms the potent health benefits of meditation. As mentioned in the Stress Management section, a meta-analysis of over 200 studies found that utilizing mediation was "especially effective" in reducing stress, depression, and anxiety,[18] which psoriasis sufferers are also often afflicted with. Research has also shown that meditation can reduce pain, symptoms of ulcerative colitis (another autoimmune disease), high blood pressure, insomnia, and other health conditions.[23] The benefits for psoriasis sufferers practicing meditation are demonstrated in research, too. One study found that those who listened to a brief guided meditation while undergoing ultraviolet light therapy experienced an increase in the rate of resolution of their psoriatic regions.[24] Our community deserves much more research on this topic.

✧ My Psoriasis Story ✧

Meditation has been, and continues to be, an incredibly healing practice for me. Meditation has given me the tools to better understand my experience while cutting through misperceptions, misunderstandings, and misguided habits. Not only have I learned how to handle stress better by using meditation, but also have found more peace surrounding my body and the feeling of a lack of control about my psoriasis.

By practicing meditation, I have come to learn what stress feels like in my body, what types of situations make me feel stressed, and also how to reduce my stress once present. It has also given me the tools and space to approach my psoriasis from a calmer perspective, as meditation encouraged me to focus on how the state of my skin does not define me as a person nor my worth. I have learned that, instead of ignoring my symptoms, by giving them attention and refining my awareness of them, then the pain becomes less scary, less foreign, and even dulls in severity. It has been a relief to work on separating my emotional self from the state of my physical body, whether good or bad. It's like stepping off a roller coaster of emotions, and constantly honing the skills to jump back off the roller coaster if and when you find yourself strapped into the seat again.

During my healing journey, I decided to first explore all that Western medicine had to offer for psoriasis sufferers, with the exception of medications, as these are just band-aids and not cures, which I was not interested in. I knew that my psoriasis was related to my gut health, but I wasn't sure how. I went to see a gastroenterologist for help in 2018. After hearing my concerns, he did admit that he didn't feel he could help me – I am still grateful for his honesty and forthrightness – and referred me instead to explore Eastern medicine. His words were ringing in my ears as I signed up for yoga teacher training, which started in January 2019. I had an appointment with a second gastroenterologist in 2019, who similarly encouraged my exploration into Eastern yogic practices. While I was familiar with meditation prior, I was about to learn much about the topic.

My first deep dive into mediation was during my yoga teacher training at Jaya Yoga Center in Brooklyn, in the spring of 2019. During this 5-month course, we had an ongoing assignment to use a meditation app regularly. We were taught various forms of meditation, such as yoga nidra. We also learned about methods of controlling the breath as meditation, known as Prāṇāyāma in Sanskrit. Variations of Prāṇāyāma that we learned included Ujjāyi (audibly exhaling with your mouth closed as if you are fogging up a window), Sama Vṛtti (equal length inhales and exhales, such as "square breathing"), Kapālabhāti (short, sharp exhalations from the diaphragm), Nāḍī Shuddhi (breathing through alternate nostrils using your fingers to close off each nostril alternately), and Nāḍī Śodhana (the same as Nāḍī Shuddhi, but with holding the breath after inhales). By the end of my yoga teacher training, a patch of psoriasis that had been on my right ankle for several years had healed completely.

I continue to learn more about Eastern healthcare practices in my exploration of Ayurveda, an ancient natural system of health and healing originating in India. Ayurveda is more than 5,000 years old, and is a Sanskrit word that translates to "the science of life and longevity."[25] I have much more to learn on these topics, and am thankful for the healing they have offered me thus far.

INTUITIVE EXERCISE

≫ GENERAL RECOMMENDATIONS ≪

Intuitive exercise is a way of viewing physical activity that centers enjoyment and the body's needs that day, while rejecting the idea that more exercise is better no matter what. It requires connecting to our body, and listening to it to figure out what type of exercise or movement it currently needs. Instead of choosing exercise based on what we think we "should" do or as "punishment" for being "bad," intuitive exercise asks us to follow our own internal cues to identify the type, length, and intensity of our workout. It also requires that we exercise for the sake of self-care or health benefits, not to abuse ourselves with negative thoughts like needing to "burn calories" or "lose weight." Ask yourself questions like: "What does my body need today?", "What type of movement do I feel like doing?", or "What type of exercise would be most beneficial to my body today?". Some days we may crave an intense workout, other days we may need just to stretch or go for a walk.[26] This mindset helps to break away from the inaccurate idea that we must exercise to balance out our food choices, also known as "calories in, calories out." In truth, the benefits of exercise are largely separate from our food habits.

This balance is critically important when working with autoimmune diseases, since there are health benefits to exercise, but health consequences to overexercising. In general, regular exercise is correlated with improved psoriasis symptoms,[27,28] however overexercising is hard on our immune system and can make our psoriasis worse. In fact, I have seen several autoimmune clients in my practice where overexercising was likely worsening or even instigating their disease state. By honing in to our bodies' needs, it can become easier to avoid overexercising and worsening our psoriasis.

If you would like more structure in this area, then the American Heart Association has some helpful recommendations for us. They suggest 150 minutes (2.5 hours) per week of moderate-intensity aerobic activity, or 75 minutes (1.25 hours) per week of vigorous aerobic activity. A combination of both moderate and vigorous intensity is also a good idea. Don't aim to meet your exercise goals in one day, and instead spread your exercises throughout the week.[29] The American College of Sports Medicine recommends strength training at least twice a week, doing 8 - 12 repetitions of 8 - 10 different exercises for each major muscle group, and stretching at least 2 - 3 days per week.[1]

I highly recommend exercise that promotes mind-body awareness, such as yoga. Seek yoga classes that emphasize calming the mind, not just intense workouts. Avoid yoga studios that have a competitive atmosphere – yoga is a life philosophy, not a competition. Traditionally, historically, and culturally, yoga is much more than just a workout – find yoga studios that honor this rich heritage.

For those who are not already in the habit of exercising, a great starting point can be to focus on walking more. One idea is to obtain a step counter (there are many step counter apps available) to get an idea of how many steps you take in a regular day. Challenge yourself to increase this number over time, perhaps until you reach the often recommended 10,000 steps per day, on average. This is equal to about 5 miles. Or, if 10,000 steps a day isn't a goal that works for you, then find the number of steps that works for you and then begin to increase the intensity of your walk. This might look like incorporating lunges, high knees, arm circles, sprints, going up and down a set of stairs, and so on. If focusing on the number of steps detracts from the enjoyment you feel, then delete the step counter app! Another suggestion is to aim for 30 minutes of movement per day, which can be broken up throughout the day. Beginning an exercise routine can be quite challenging, but in time you will be shocked to discover how much you have come to enjoy it.

• • • MORE ON THE SCIENCE • • •

In general, regular exercise is correlated with improved psoriasis symptoms.[27,28] Exercising positively affects our microbiome,[30] improves our mood, reduces our risk of heart disease (a common comorbidity for psoriasis sufferers), improves cognitive functioning, improves sleep quality, and so much more.[31] Getting adequate exercise is important for its stress-reducing and also cardioprotective properties, both of which are especially important for folks with psoriasis. All of this better prepares us to handle – and heal from – our psoriasis.

However, even too much of a good thing can be a bad thing, and overexercising can prevent our psoriasis from improving. Overexercising is damaging because it stimulates the fight-or-flight nervous system, which in turn suppresses the immune system.

Activities such as prolonged intensive exercise, high exercise training workloads, competitive events, intensive endurance exercise, and the like are associated with immune dysfunction, inflammation, and oxidative stress[27] – all of which may exacerbate an autoimmune condition. So, do exercise – but not too much.

✧ MY PSORIASIS STORY ✧

Getting enough movement – but not too much! – is a balance I'm constantly looking to strike. It's all about constant readjustments, and keeping an eye on my body and habits. If I notice that one week I've been moving less, then I will aim to get more activity in the next week. If I've been exercising so much that I'm starting to feel exhausted and drained by it – well, then it's time to cut down.

I keep active by walking my dog for 30 - 60 minutes on weekday mornings, and biking to work 2 - 3 days per week (about 40 minutes total of biking per day). Often my partner and I will carve out time during our weekend to go hiking, play handball, throw around a basketball, work out in the park, or simply go on a walk in a new place. If I need to cut down on exercise, I will drive or take the bus to work instead of biking.

I never count calories "burned" and rarely keep track of the total time I spend exercising per week, but instead focus on how I'm feeling and what I know. If I know I haven't been moving much and my body feels stiff and achy, it's time to get out there. If I know I've been moving a lot and my body tires quickly, then I can lay off for a bit.

AIR POLLUTION

≫ GENERAL RECOMMENDATIONS ≪

Reducing the amount of air pollutants we inhale can have a huge impact on our psoriasis. Everything from cigarette smoke to household mold to car traffic should be on your radar. If you do smoke cigarettes or otherwise, clearly the best thing to do for your psoriasis (and overall health, too) would be to quit, or at least don't smoke indoors. If you suspect that indoor mold may be present in high levels in your home, it may be wise to speak to an expert about the severity of the issue and options for remediation.

If you live in a major city or near a heavily used road or highway, you may want to consider purchasing a HEPA air filter and running it regularly in your home to improve air quality. If you are unable to avoid air pollution, like those of us who live in large cities, then consider purchasing and wearing an N95 mask while outside, especially when you are exercising vigorously outdoors. This mask will filter out any air pollution particles larger than 0.3 microns. This frees up your lungs from having to do the heavy work of removing these pollutants from your body by never breathing them in in the first place.

··· MORE ON THE SCIENCE ···

Exposure to air pollution is associated with psoriasis, as it can severely interfere with the normal functioning of fatty acids, DNA, and/or proteins that make up our skin via oxidative damage. Even cigarette smoke is associated with psoriasis.[32] Cadmium, a heavy metal, is another air pollutant associated with psoriasis, as it is a ubiquitous environmental contaminant and is toxic even at low levels. One study over almost 6,000 participants found that those with severe psoriasis also had higher blood cadmium, and exposure to cadmium can predispose someone to having worse psoriasis. Usually, someone would be exposed to cadmium through tobacco smoke, food (main sources being cereals and vegetables), contaminated air and dust near industrial sites and main roads, or at their job (cadmium is used in pigments, batteries, plating and coatings, plastic stabilizers, photovoltaic devices, nonferrous alloys, and more). Cadmium can increase the risk of multiple-organ disease and metabolic syndrome. Cadmium also causes the elevation of inflammation markers and negatively influences the immune system. It appears that cadmium accumulation can affect psoriasis through various ways, such as through oxidative stress, cadmium-induced zinc deficiency, changes in immune response, and upregulation inflammation markers.[33] Air pollution has been linked to the development of autoimmune diseases in general.[34,35,36]

While I'm unable to find research specific to this topic, there are several stories out there in the psoriasis community of folks who discovered that household mold was promoting or causing their psoriasis. People have recounted how they moved into a new home and suddenly experienced a large flare-up of psoriasis, often which doesn't resolve until they remediate the mold or move out of that house. There should absolutely be research conducted on this topic.

✧ My Psoriasis Story ✧

Air pollution definitely impacts my psoriasis, and it only took a global pandemic for me to learn this. While the COVID-19 pandemic has been (and still is, at the time of this writing) an entirely awful and tragic series of events, there has been a silver lining for me. I was living in Brooklyn when COVID hit New York City, and watched firsthand as this virus ravaged my once-flourishing city. The summer streets that used to be filled with music, laughter, and the clink of dishes at nearby restaurants devolved into silence, only broken by ambulance sirens several times a day.

During this time, the usual constant flow of traffic slowed dramatically. We drove effortlessly through Manhattan at what would have been rush hour, except there was no traffic at all. The highway near my house emptied. The roads were quiet. And the air started to smell different, to feel lighter in my nose. My partner and I both commented on how much different the air smelt and felt, and could easily attribute it to the reduction in car traffic. The change was so obvious we couldn't miss it.

A few months before COVID hit, I went to the ENT (a doctor for your ear, nose, and throat – also called an otolaryngologist). For years I was constantly clearing my throat, as there was always an irritating tickle back there. I was chronically congested. I felt like I couldn't smell very well. I wondered if these symptoms were related to my psoriasis. The ENT diagnosed me with chronic rhinitis, said the mucus in my nose was unusually thick and probably irritating to my throat via post-nasal drip, then referred me to an allergist. The allergist did some skin allergy tests, and found a few moderate allergies to cats, dogs, cockroaches, and a few plants. Both doctors offered steroid nasal sprays. I was reminded of when I went to a dermatologist in 2018, who offered me a topical steroid cream. Steroids didn't feel like an answer, just a band-aid. I left these doctor's' offices with some more information, but no clear answers. I considered doing allergy shots, in the hopes that they would help my psoriasis, but ended up not following through due to the COVID pandemic.

During those few weeks when the traffic almost disappeared, all of the symptoms I went to the ENT and allergist for suddenly evaporated. My throat was no longer itchy. I was relieved of my throat clearing. My sense of smell was stronger. I no longer felt congested. Ah ha – air pollution was my problem! Of course, it made so much sense. I bought a HEPA air filter in the summer of 2020, I began using it every night, and soon after my psoriasis went into remission for the first time in 6.5 years.

Now, I try to sleep every night with the HEPA air filter running. It was adding this filter to my life, on top of all of the other changes I had made, that pushed me into remission. When I forget to use it regularly, my psoriasis begins to flare up again, like clockwork.

Also, when I bike around the city and will be breathing heavily near car exhaust pipes, I wear an N-95 mask. This mask filters out any air pollution particles larger than 0.3 microns. These two measures have been quite helpful in managing, reducing, and ultimately putting my psoriasis into remission.

As mentioned in the Benefits of Fasting section, the connection between air quality and my psoriasis became apparent again during my trip in September 2020 to visit family in Colorado. While I was in town, one of the largest wildfires in Colorado history was raging to the northwest of us, plus there were record-breaking fires in California, Oregon, and Washington also burning. The air quality index (AQI) often hovered around "Unhealthy" to "Hazardous." We kept a HEPA air filter running 24 hours a day in the house, which helped, but alone it wasn't enough, and my psoriasis flared up again. Even though I had previously been in complete remission, now all of a sudden my belly button, elbows, and ankles burst open with new psoriasis spots. It used to be that my psoriasis reliably *improved* while on vacation, which I came to learn was because my stress levels dropped significantly on vacation. Now I was experiencing the opposite, so it was quite clear that poor air quality caused my flare-up during this vacation.

While of course I wish COVID had never happened or at least had been better contained early, I am still thankful for this incredibly powerful lesson that it taught me.

SLEEP

≫ GENERAL RECOMMENDATIONS ≪

Getting enough (or extra!) sleep is very important to healing psoriasis. The amount of hours we should sleep in a day varies by our age. For the majority of adults (ages 18 - 64), 7 - 9 hours is recommended. For those over 65 years old, 7 - 8 hours is the goal, and children 6 - 13 years old should aim for 9 - 11 hours a night.[37] In my personal experience, times when I can sleep even more than the recommended amount have been met with increased psoriasis healing.

If you have trouble sleeping, there are many natural ways to promote sleep that may be beneficial. Possibly the most helpful is to get more exercise; although it may take several days of increased physical activity levels before you start joyously yawning around bedtime. If anxiety or racing thoughts are keeping you up, it may help to relax by trying a magnesium supplement, CBD, or adaptogens (particularly ashwagandha). Taking even just one minute to meditate before bed can also make a big difference – see the Meditation section for further guidance. There are some foods that are important to avoid, as well – such as excessive alcohol or caffeine in the afternoon and later, as these can also disrupt your sleep.

Another strategy to promote sleep is to work on your sleep hygiene. This includes keeping a stable bedtime and wake-up time, making your bedroom comfortable and free from distractions or work, following the same pre-bedtime routine each night, keep the lights dim near bedtime, and avoid screens for at least 30 - 60 minutes before bedtime.[38]

If you suffer from sleep apnea or experience snoring, recurrent awakening during sleep, and excessive daytime sleepiness, it is recommended that you consult with a lung doctor (called a respirologist or pulmonologist) and/or have a sleep study done.[39] Depression is another condition that can exacerbate sleep problems – consult with a medical provider such as a psychologist or psychiatrist to assist with managing depression.

• • • MORE ON THE SCIENCE • • •

Getting adequate sleep is one way we can promote proper circadian rhythm functioning. This is discussed in depth in the Benefits of Eating Regularly section, but the highlights are that a healthy, regular circadian rhythm is important for long-term health and that higher rates of psoriasis are seen in people who have a disrupted circadian rhythm, such as night-shift workers.

That said, it can be harder for psoriasis sufferers to get enough sleep, as we tend to suffer from higher rates of fatigue[40] and insomnia, plus psoriasis itself may keep us awake[41] with itching, soreness, and pain. Unfortunately, this puts us at a significantly higher risk for cardiovascular disease.[42] It's interesting to note that one study found that "Fatigue severity was associated with smoking, pain and depression, but not with psoriasis severity."[40] Additionally, psoriasis sufferers tend to have higher rates of sleep apnea, as a recent meta-analysis has concluded. The analysis noted that medical practitioners should ask their psoriatic patients about their sleep quality. Psoriasis sufferers with night snoring, recurrent awaking, and excessive daytime sleepiness should consult with a respirologist/pulmonologist and/or have a polysomnography (sleep study) done.[39]

✧ MY PSORIASIS STORY ✧

The connection between good sleep quality and our overall physical and mental health is undeniable. I work regularly with my clients to improve their sleep quality. For myself, it's critical that I get around 8 hours of sleep each night. In fact, I notice that I almost always wake up about 8 hours after I fall asleep, no matter what time I fall asleep, so it's clear to see that my body prefers this amount of sleep.

When my psoriasis first started developing in college, I definitely was not getting enough sleep, I had poor sleep hygiene, and also no reliable sleep schedule. This was one of my least favorite parts of college: the erratic schedule. Our bodies thrive off of schedules, and the lack of a schedule contributed to the development of my psoriasis.

Once I graduated and began working regular hours, thankfully I was able to return to a consistent schedule of sleeping, working, and eating. Improvements in my sleep pattern have always come at the same time as other lifestyle improvements, so it's hard for me to tease out the effects of inadequate sleep on my psoriasis, but I have no doubt at all that sleep is incredibly important to the healing process.

I am still working on improving my sleep hygiene now. Since I suffer from anxiety, it can be quite difficult for me to lay in bed trying to fall asleep, as my mind starts racing about all of the stuff I need to get done and my worries. I use watching TV as a crutch to avoid these racings thoughts before bed – but sometimes fall asleep on the couch or have vivid dreams related to the show, which do not help my sleep quality. I'm working on weaning myself off of falling asleep in front of the TV. Currently, I allow myself to watch TV until tiredness starts to tug at my eyelids, then I try to go to bed immediately. This requires that, before I watch TV, everything is ready (my phone is plugged in, I've gone to the bathroom and brushed my teeth, I'm in my PJs, my water bottle is on my nightstand, etc) so I can jump straight into bed once I begin to get tired. If I wake up on the couch and, for example, need to plug my phone in before getting into bed, then that will wake me up too much so I can't fall back asleep. At times, I can avoid watching TV all together by meditating before going to bed. I just recently set an alarm with a soothing tone to go off at 9pm every night, which is my reminder that it's time to start getting ready for bed.

One strategy that almost always helps me to fall asleep quicker and also improves my sleep quality is meditating for even just a minute around my bedtime. However, even though I know it's extremely helpful for me, meditating before bed is something I struggle to do regularly. To help myself meditate more often before bed, recently I have been encouraging myself to meditate on my breathing during the commercials when I watch TV before bed. If I meditate over a few commercial breaks, I notice that it's easier to fall into a calm, restful sleep.

I continue to work on improving my sleep quality.

Dogs & Other Pets

≫ General Recommendations ≪

If you've been thinking about getting a dog, now may be the time! Dogs are particularly helpful pets because they generally require that we take them on regular walks, which increases our physical activity levels and promotes joint health for those of us who have experienced psoriatic arthritis. Dog ownership is associated with a lower rate of death in general, and a lower risk of heart disease particularly if you live alone.[43] Other pets can be helpful, too, as simply petting animals is associated with reducing anxiety.[44] Dogs may also help to improve the health of our skin microbiome, which is disordered in psoriasis sufferers.

• • • More on the Science • • •

The main benefits of dog ownership for the psoriasis sufferer are reduced risk of overall mortality and heart disease, increased exercise levels, social and emotional support, lower levels of stress and anxiety, plus improved joint health. A 12-year nation-wide study of over 3 million people in Sweden found a reduced risk of death from cardiovascular disease (CVD) plus other causes of death in dog owners, and an even lower risk of CVD for those living alone. Those who owned hunting breed dogs had the lowest risk of CVD.[45] With psoriasis sufferers more likely to experience CVD and with CVD being the leading cause of death worldwide (excluding pandemics, as the coronavirus global pandemic still runs rampant at the time of this writing), this is a substantial benefit. This study proposes that the two main ways that dog ownership supports health is by increasing exercise levels and by providing social and emotional support.

Dog ownership can encourage us to be more physically active, which of course is generally associated with improved health outcomes. This can be helpful for psoriatic arthritis as well. Since about one-third of psoriasis sufferers will go on to develop psoriatic arthritis, moderate exercise is important as it can help with decreasing joint pain, inflammation, and stiffness while increasing range of motion.[46] Animals can also provide social and emotional support. Research shows that petting animals can reduce anxiety levels.[44] Folks with severe psoriasis may feel socially isolated and excluded, due to the shame and embarrassment of suffering from such a visible disease[47] that strangers often misunderstand, and having an animal companion can reduce these negative feelings.

Additionally, there may be another benefit to dog ownership for psoriasis sufferers. Research demonstrates that the skin microbiome on psoriatic lesions is significantly disrupted. Some studies have demonstrated that psoriatic areas have increased microbial diversity compared to healthy skin, and other studies have shown a decreased microbial diversity. In short, the skin microbiome is largely disordered in psoriatic areas.[48] Therefore, it may prove helpful to find ways to support a balanced, stable, healthy skin microbiome. Research has established that the skin microbiome of the people we live with affects our skin microbiome and visa versa, especially for couples. Dogs expedite this process, as they significantly increase the skin microbiota that humans share. Plus, dog owners also share skin microbiota with their dog itself.[49] In this way, it's possible that having a dog may promote a healthier skin microbiome that is less likely to develop psoriasis. Furthermore, it's also possible that if you live with someone who doesn't have psoriasis, dogs may also facilitate spreading their healthier skin microbiome to you. However, a note of caution as in theory this may also make it easier to spread the less healthy psoriasis microbiome to household members who don't currently have psoriasis. While I was unable to find research specifically on this topic, this is a plausible hypothesis that deserves further research.

✧ MY PSORIASIS STORY ✧

While I already love dogs and wanted to get a dog just for the fun of it, psoriasis was absolutely on my mind when we decided to adopt our little Frida doggie from Animal Care Centers of NYC, a nearby animal shelter. I had heard that dogs could help improve microbiome diversity, and knew that was something I could use some help with. After a few adorable licks to the face, Frida came home with us on a crisp sunny day in November 2019.

Even though during my visit to the allergist (more on this in the Reduce Exposure to Air Pollution section) I tested as slightly allergic to dogs, I felt that if I was exposed to a dog regularly then my canine allergies would subside. I grew up with dogs and felt my sensitivity to them increase the longer I lived without one, so I felt fairly certain about my hypothesis. Luckily, I was right. The first few weeks with Frida my allergies flared up – I was itchy and even more congested than normal – and right when I was afraid that I might get sick from all the irritation, things began to calm down. The itching subsided, and my congestion reduced back to baseline.

It's hard to tease out the exact effect that getting a dog has had, but I definitely believe that she has positively impacted my psoriasis. Frida helps keep my physical activity levels up, as I take her on long walks in the morning almost everyday. I've found that these walks are good for my stress levels, and it's beneficial for my mental health to get out of the house early in the day. During the worst of the COVID pandemic here in NYC, she was my constant companion (since my partner was deemed an "essential worker," but unable to work remotely, and had to go to work everyday), and she reminded me to get out of the house and eat regularly. I attribute what remains intact of my sanity during this pandemic to Frida's presence. Plus, just petting and snuggling her all the time brings a lot of joy and peace to my life.

△ △ △ △

Additional Thoughts

"According to Ayurveda, health is not simply the absence of disease. It is rather a state of balance among body, mind, and consciousness."

— Vasant Lad, BAMS MASc,
founder of the Ayurvedic Institute and author of
The Complete Book of Ayurvedic Home Remedies

△ △ △ △

The below is a compilation of psoriasis-related information and thoughts that arose during my research that does not fit into the five strategies, but may still be of interest to you. These are listed in no particular order.

Hormones & Pregnancy

Hormones and the hormonal shifts that occur during pregnancy can have an interesting effect on psoriasis. If you plan to get pregnant, then know that frequently pregnancy is accompanied by an improvement in symptoms. Some people even report that they went into complete remission while pregnant. One study of 47 pregnant psoriasis sufferers found that 55% experienced improvement while pregnant, 21% reported no change, and 23% reported that their symptoms got worse. The authors of this study concluded that the high levels of the hormone estrogen seen during pregnancy were correlated with improvement in psoriasis. Estrogen has both immunosuppressive and immunostimulatory properties. Levels of the hormone progesterone also rise during pregnancy, but this wasn't correlated with psoriasis changes in this study. The authors also mention reports from psoriasis sufferers that their skin worsens when estrogen and progesterone levels drop, such as after birth, before their period starts, and at menopause.[1]

THE ANTIBIOTICS & ANTIFUNGALS QUESTION

Increasing our understanding of psoriasis and the microbiome – which antibiotics and antifungals directly impact – is one of the current frontiers in psoriasis research. There is a definite correlation between psoriasis and the microbiome, particularly our skin and intestinal microbiomes.[2,3,4] However, what to do with this information is really the question, and at the moment it is a controversial topic because there are no clear answers.[5] I have no doubt that taking antibiotics triggered the worst psoriasis of my life – it didn't act alone though; instead it was the straw that broke the camel's back (see the Introduction to My Psoriasis Story section for more on this) – and so I have been very tempted to recommend that other folks with psoriasis also avoid antibiotics. In my case, I believe that taking antibiotics allowed an infection of the fungus *Candida albicans* to grow (more on this in the Sugar section). Yet, broadly avoiding antibiotics isn't supported by research. I wish I knew exactly which antibiotics I took, however I no longer have those records.

This is what the current research does have to say on the topic of antibiotics. One study from the United Kingdom of 845 children 15 years old and younger with newly developed psoriasis found only a weak link between antibiotics exposure and psoriasis development.[6] Previous case reports and observational studies linked the antibiotic tetracycline to psoriasis development.[6] Conversely, two other studies found improvements in psoriasis from long-term antibiotic regimens. One study of 30 patients with moderate to severe chronic plaque psoriasis were given the antibiotic azithromycin over 48 weeks. At the end of 48 weeks, 18 patients (60%) showed excellent improvement, 6 patients (20%) showed good improvement, and 4 patients (13.33%) showed mild improvement (2 patients did not complete the study). After following up on the patients 1 year later, they found that 6 patients (20%) experienced a recurrence of psoriasis.[7] A second study gave 30 psoriatic patients the antibiotic benzathine penicillin over 48 weeks. The researchers reported that all the patients showed excellent improvement at 2 years.[8] Both of these studies suggest that some psoriatic folks may have subclinical streptococcal infections that the antibiotics cleared up.[7,8]

The story continues with antifungal drugs. Levels of the fungus *Candida albicans* are significantly higher in psoriatic folks,[4] and researchers suggest that "antifungal treatment should be considered as an adjuvant treatment of psoriasis."[3] While I chose to get my *Candida* overgrowth under control naturally by using antifungal herbs, foods, and teas (more on my regimen in the My Psoriasis Story in the Sugar section), antifungal drugs may prove to have a significant benefit to some psoriasis sufferers. I will also note that one of the main supplements I used to get my *Candida* infection under control was oregano oil, which has not only antibacterial, but also antifungal and antiviral properties. This was possibly more beneficial for my system than exclusively taking a prescribed antibiotic or antifungal.

Personally, since I've already had an extremely negative experience with them, I still choose to steer clear of most man-made antibiotic products. I used hand sanitizer in between every single patient when I worked in a hospital per sanitation protocols, and I've used some hand sanitizer during the COVID pandemic – but otherwise I stay away from antibacterial drugs, soaps, cleaners, fabrics, surfaces, chemicals, and so on. That's the decision I have made for now that feels right to me, but may not be the best decision for all psoriasis sufferers.

Drug Induced & Provoked Psoriasis

There are some drugs that have been associated with either initiating or exacerbating psoriasis. At this point in time, "although well-conducted systematic studies on drug-related psoriasis are mostly lacking,"[9] associations have been documented for:

- Nonsteroidal anti-inflammatory drugs (NSAIDs) (Indomethacin [Tivorbex] and naproxen [Aleve] - oral naproxen is the most associated with psoriasis exacerbation).
- Beta-blockers (Atenolol [Tenormin], metoprolol [Lopressor, Toprol XL], propranolol [Hemangeol, Inderal, InnoPran XL])
- Antibiotic tetracycline
- Some mental health medications (Lithium, alprazolam [Niravam, Xanax], clonazepam [Klonopin], diazepam [Valium])
- Some heart medications (Amiodarone, digoxin [Lanoxicaps, Lanoxin], gemfibrozil [Lopid], quinidine)
- Antimalarial drugs (chloroquine [Aralen] and hydroxychloroquine [Plaquenil])
- Interferons
- Imiquimod
- Terbinafine (Lamisil, Terbinex)
- Angiotensin-converting enzyme (ACE) inhibitors
- Benzodiazepines
- Clonidine
- Gold
- TNF-α inhibitors
- Fluoxetine
- Cimetidine.[5,9,10]

Discuss further with a medical doctor to best understand whether these medications should be avoided or not for you.

POTENTIAL BENEFITS OF A TONSILLECTOMY

Autoimmune conditions are often described as having an "overactive" immune system, so it may come as no surprise that physically removing part of our immune system can help reduce psoriasis symptoms. Removing the tonsils – a tonsillectomy – "can be an effective treatment for palmoplantar pustulosis, plaque psoriasis, and guttate psoriasis." However, the strength of this evidence is in question, as most of the studies are limited to case reports and case series. One randomized trial of 29 patients with plaque psoriasis "showed a significant benefit to tonsillectomy that was sustained over a two-year follow-up period."[11]

AVOIDING STREP THROAT & PROMOTING THROAT HEALTH

Strep (*Streptococcus*) throat infections are a well known common trigger for psoriasis.[12,13] Strep throat infections have "been shown to be a significant trigger of psoriasis in some patients, possibly by sensitizing T cells to keratin epitopes in the skin."[11] Furthermore, folks with psoriasis have been found to get strep throat infections 10 times more frequently than those without psoriasis![13] To me, the next logical question is what we can do in our daily lives to prevent a strep infection.

There are several strategies that I personally use to maintain throat health. I run a portable HEPA air filter in my house everyday and I use a neti pot (also called "nasal irrigation") regularly, which significantly reduces my congestion. Both of these help to reduce the chronic throat clearing I experience otherwise (more on both of these topics in the Reduce Exposure to Air Pollution section). However, to my knowledge these strategies are not necessarily supported by research as prevention against strep throat or other throat infections, and I can only offer them as my personal experience. I also find it very important to keep up with brushing and flossing my teeth regularly, so an infection has a lower chance of growing. Interestingly, there is one Scandinavian study that found that the prevalence of gum disease is 24% higher in folks with psoriasis,[14] although the researchers did not relate this back to strep throat. When I feel like I may be brewing a throat infection, I mix up a mason jar of salt water with a splash of apple cider vinegar, and gargle it multiple times a day. Gargling salt water is a well-known home remedy for strep throat or any sore throat,[15] and I like to use it preventatively when I feel that I am starting to get a sore throat.

The first and last time I know for sure that I had a strep infection was in 10th grade. I was so sick that I ended up with two infections – strep throat and the flu. It is around that time that my mom and I remember my psoriasis starting and, if memory serves, after I recovered is when I started to develop small transient patches on my elbows. I feel that this episode promoted the development of my psoriasis, and set the stage for my psoriasis to worsen over time.

TOXINS & HEAVY METAL EXPOSURE

Another potential issue with psoriasis sufferers may be heavy metal toxicity. One study of 5,927 participants found that psoriatic patients had significantly higher blood levels of the heavy metal cadmium. The researchers also found higher levels of cadmium to be linearly associated with an increase in psoriasis severity. Exposure to cadmium is usually through smoking and food. Cereals and vegetables are the main source of dietary cadmium in humans. Living near areas with contaminated air and dust, like near major roads and industrial sites, pose another important potential exposure risk. It appears that cadmium accumulation can affect psoriasis through various ways, such as through oxidative stress, cadmium-induced zinc deficiency, changes in immune response, and upregulation of inflammation markers.[16] Avoiding continued exposure to cadmium may help to naturally increase your zinc levels, and ultimately help ease psoriasis severity. One meta-analysis of 15 studies found that decreased blood levels of zinc were generally observed in patients with psoriasis.[17] Since conventionally grown grains can be a source of cadmium, I wonder if those who find relief from following a diet that removes grains (like the Paleo or the Autoimmune Protocol [AIP] diets) may be inadvertently treating high cadmium levels. Choosing organically grown foods whenever possible is recommended, as organic crops are found to have lower levels of cadmium while boasting higher levels of antioxidants.[18]

Another potentially helpful strategy is to reduce our exposure to other "toxins" in general. While the role of environmental toxins is a topic that could fill another book, I will refer to a popular book on another autoimmune disease – Hashimoto's Protocol by Dr. Izabella Wentz – to briefly address this multifaceted subject matter. Dr. Wentz recommends:

- Avoiding antibacterial products, especially triclosan. If you must disinfect, use alcohol.
- Cooking in/with and eating off of glass, ceramic, cast iron, wooden utensils, and parchment paper. Avoid plastic, stainless steel, Teflon, and aluminum foil.
- Getting an air purifier. This should help to improve poor air quality which may result from off-gassing building materials, VOCs, airborne pathogens, pollens, and molds.
- Going without personal care products or reducing your regimen as much as possible. This includes make-up, nail polish, lotion, shampoo, make-up remover, face masks, hair spray, perfume, and so on. Toxins from topical products can be absorbed at a higher rate than if we ate them!
- Increasing sweating and fiber intake, to support the body in removing toxins.[19]

Since sweating is one of the ways that the body naturally removes toxins, I recommend using natural deodorants that do not contain antiperspirants, as antiperspirants impede the body's ability to sweat. Mold testing in your home may be another prudent measure. Whenever possible, purchasing organic foods is an additional way we can reduce our toxin exposure, as pesticide exposure is increasingly being correlated with autoimmune diseases.[20,21]

Again, this is a vast topic that is not covered in full here. The impacts of these innumerable toxins on psoriasis has yet to be fully illuminated by research.

CHRONIC SUBACUTE INFECTIONS

It has been noted that people with psoriasis may suffer from low-grade chronic infections that are serious enough to take a toll on our health, but not severe enough to be clearly evident (also called latent, subacute, or subclinical infections). An example of this is *Candida albicans* (often referred to as simply "*Candida*"), which is outlined in depth in the Sugar section. Another example is strep throat (*Streptococcus pyogenes*), as described in the Avoiding Strep Throat section. Another such possible subacute infection is *H. pylori* (*Helicobacter pylori*).[22] Ask your doctor if they will evaluate you further and test for these infections.

Finally, it's worth noting that at least at this time it appears that Lyme disease and viruses in the herpes family (including chickenpox, shingles, Epstein-Barr virus [aka "mono"], and more) are NOT associated with psoriasis.[23]

THE QUESTION OF ZINC

While zinc is known for its positive impact on the immune system, at this time there is no evidence that supplementing with zinc is helpful for reducing psoriasis. In a controlled double-blind study with twenty-five psoriatic patients, who were given either an oral zinc supplementation or placebo over 12 weeks, there were no statistically significant changes in the psoriasis area or severity.[24] Interestingly, however, when compared to the general population, people with psoriasis have significantly decreased serum zinc levels (and also significantly increased serum copper levels).[17] It's possible that this low zinc status could be caused by heavy metal toxicity, such as cadmium, as discussed above in the Toxins &

Heavy Metal Exposure section. Reducing exposure to cadmium may prove to be more helpful than supplementing with zinc.

However, topically applied zinc has been used as a psoriasis treatment. A randomized double-blind controlled trial found that topical 0.25% zinc pyrithione cream, applied twice daily, is effective for localized plaque psoriasis.[25]

Hydration

While I'm unable to find any research on the topic, it's not uncommon for people in psoriasis support groups and forums to mention that staying well hydrated is important to reducing their psoriasis severity. It makes sense, too, since psoriatic skin gets so dry and cracked, so drinking more water would help keep the skin more moisturized. The general recommendation is to drink eight 8-ounce glasses, which equals about 2 liters or half a gallon, per day. You can and should include any other fluids you ingest in this total too, such as tea, coffee, soup, and milk. It may be best to drink filtered water. Again, much more research is needed in this area.

The Lasting Impacts of Trauma

Traumatic experiences, across the lifespan, have been associated with psoriasis development. In a study of 100 psoriatic patients and 101 controls, "negative traumatic experiences appeared more frequently in patients with psoriasis during all developmental periods." Interestingly, "no correlation between severity of psoriasis and traumatic experiences" has been noted.[26] Another study of 27 psoriasis patients and 26 controls showed that people with psoriasis have a "significant prevalence of childhood trauma and a lower resilience level compared to healthy controls."[27]

△ △ △ △

A NOTE ON "OBESITY" &
WEIGHT STIGMA

"Cultural fatphobia predates any health
arguments about body size."

— Christy Harrison, MPH, RD, CDN,
Intuitive Eating Coach and Anti-Diet Dietitian

△ △ △ △

A common food-related concern among medical doctors treating psoriasis, such as primary care doctors, dermatologists, and rheumatologists, is the weight status of their patients. When they are treating patients who are considered "overweight" or "obese," these specialists may recommend losing weight as a way to reduce psoriasis severity. However, the effectiveness and appropriateness of these recommendations is now rightfully being questioned.

First, long-term weight loss is rarely achieved, as research demonstrates that five years after a significant weight loss, more than 80% of people regained the weight they initially lost.[1] Additionally, health practitioners can have internal biases against those they perceive as overweight and inaccurately attribute negative personality traits to that person, such as thinking that their patient is lazy, stupid, or worthless.[2] This can be incredibly detrimental to the quality of treatment these patients receive, and damage the patient's psychological health.

Furthermore, it is well known in the dietetics community that the metric used to determine weight status, BMI (or body mass index), is based on suboptimal science. The BMI calculation was created by Belgian mathematician Lambert Adolphe Jacques Quetelet in the early 1800s, who explicitly stated "that it could not and should not be used to indicate the level of fatness in an individual."[3] BMI does not take into account differences in muscle mass, bone mass, fat mass, waist circumference, gender, ethnicity/race, or age,[3,4,5,6,7] making its reliability – or lack of – to be of great concern. To complicate things even more, "mild obesity" is actually associated with an improved survival rate,[8] and "about a third of people with normal BMI measures [have] an unhealthy cardiometabolic profile."[9] It begs the question – is having a larger body alone responsible for the commonly associated negative health consequences, or does the stigma and discrimination that comes along with living in a larger body promote these health concerns? Hayley Miller, a fellow dietitian nutritionist and psychotherapist who specializes in treating eating disorders, explains that "at the end of the day we don't know enough about causation when it comes to autoimmune and other diseases like cancer to see the exact correlation between weight alone and disease incidence." Teasing out the intricacies between the negative health impacts of being "overweight" versus the emotional and physical burden of being discriminated against for being a larger person will require much more future research and inquiry.[10,11]

However, something quite clear is that larger bodies and eating disorders can occur together. In fact, some researchers are even calling to merge the fields of obesity and eating disorders, as fat shaming and internalized fat bias can lead to the development of an eating disorder.[12] Since autoimmune diseases are bidirectionally correlated with eating disorders,[13,14,15] it's absolutely critical that the arguments against using BMI and inaccurately classifying people as "overweight" or "obese" are taken very seriously.

Not only does the rampant anti-fat bias in our healthcare system jeopardize the mental health of psoriasis sufferers, but is also poorly supported by research. In studies on mice, researchers found that specific food components exacerbated psoriasis rather than having a higher weight itself.[16] Additionally, "it is difficult to show what comes first, psoriasis or obesity. Pronounced social isolation, poor eating habits, depression, increased alcohol consumption, and decreased physical activity in patients with psoriasis might explain how psoriasis might lead to obesity."[16] Exposure to anti-fat bias may exacerbate these risk factors. Psoriasis is also characterized by chronic inflammation.[16] Being at a higher weight is also associated with increased pro-inflammatory markers, in particular cytokine tumor necrosis factor alpha (TNF-α)[17,18] which is also elevated in psoriasis.[19] This may at least in part explain why "obesity" is considered an independent risk factor for psoriasis.[16,20] The relationship between psoriasis and larger bodies is theorized to be bidirectional, "with obesity predisposing to psoriasis and psoriasis favoring obesity."[18] Instead of obsessing over weight, what is most important is to address the underlying risk factors.

Focusing on the strategies outlined in this book are much more useful than focusing on weight alone. Additionally, making these types of eating pattern and lifestyle changes may contribute to weight loss anyway – but they don't *have* to cause weight loss in order to be effective. Improving your eating pattern and lifestyle will likely improve your psoriasis and promote overall longevity *whether or not* it also causes weight loss. Ms. Miller explains this further: "If you're supposed to be a higher weight, then your body will work efficiently and protect you from disease rather than increase the incidence of disease." It's important to remember that our bodies *want* to be healthy, and that may look like existing in a larger body. As a result, it is unsafe for a medical practitioner to recommend weight loss alone instead of addressing underlying factors, especially for psoriasis sufferers. In my work as a dietitian nutritionist, I absolutely never encourage my clients to obsess over weight loss, and instead I alway focus our discussion on strategies that will certainly improve overall health, such as increasing fruit and vegetable intake. It's also notable that, in online psoriasis forums and support groups, it is commonly discussed how losing weight did NOT help to reduce people's psoriasis. For more information on these topics, please explore the Health at Every Size (HAES) and intuitive eating movements.

△ △ △ △

Conclusion

"A physician, though well versed in the knowledge and treatment of disease, who does not enter into the heart of the patient with the virtue of light and love, will not be able to heal the patient."

— Charaka,
Ancient Indian physician and one of the
founders of Ayurvedic medicine

△ △ △ △

To the best of my knowledge at the time of this writing, this is the first evidence-based book written on the topic of eating patterns, lifestyle, and psoriasis. It has been my honor and pleasure to draw these connections between the research world and bring them more clearly into the light of the public view. Since I suffer from psoriasis myself and have found an incredible amount of healing through changes in my eating pattern and lifestyle, I feel almost a moral imperative to support and inform my community in this way. I have attended medical conventions on psoriasis packed to the brim with medical doctors – yet heard zero information on the types of high-quality research I cite in this book. If you peruse psoriasis forums across the internet, there are massive threads overflowing with psoriasis sufferers seeking alternative options to the intense prescription medications. It's shocking how desperate the psoriasis community wants this information – and even though the research supports alternative measures such as dietary and lifestyle changes to manage psoriasis – this information does not seem to make it into doctors' clinics nearly enough.

While writing this book, I was pleasantly surprised by the amount of research already available to support my work, yet I hope I still made it abundantly clear that much more research needs to be done on these topics. Many of the studies I cited would benefit from being replicated, in order to support and strengthen the significance of their findings. Regardless, the research as it currently stands already demonstrates that eating patterns and lifestyle are very promising natural treatment modalities for psoriasis sufferers.

If you are already working with a dermatologist or rheumatologist or plan to make an appointment with one, I encourage you to ask them what their thoughts are on the impact of food and lifestyle on this disease process – however, prepare yourself to hear misinformation. If it is within your comfort level, support our community by requesting that they refer other psoriatic patients to a dietitian nutritionist who specializes in autoimmune diseases instead of recommending dietary changes themselves.

I sincerely hope from the bottom of my heart that you find a great deal of healing from this book, and can utilize these strategies for years to come to reduce your psoriasis severity. My goal is for your psoriasis flares to be small, predictable, manageable, and short-lived – and ideally to even go into remission naturally. May our psoriasis community continue to find answers, heal ourselves, and support each other well into the future!

✧ CONCLUSION TO MY PSORIASIS STORY ✧

It was 2012 when my psoriasis became a notable, significant, and persistent problem in my life. I set out on this journey to identify what exactly was causing this to happen to my body, and years of research finally led me into full remission 6.5 years later, in June of 2020. I was able to maintain remission until September of the same year, when I went on a trip to my home state of Colorado. At the time, Colorado was experiencing record-breaking and devastating forest fires. The air quality was so poor that it was scary, and my psoriasis flared up once again while on vacation.

Once I returned home to NYC, I was hoping to quickly go back into remission, but I wasn't quite so lucky. I had trouble healing again because many of my triggers were present. Stress levels were high as I continued to survive through the COVID-19 pandemic, plus the highly contentious 2020 presidential election. Soon after this, my birthday came along in late November and I was consuming sugar, gluten, and alcohol at levels that – while enjoyable and without regret – were too high to let my psoriasis heal again. Then I discovered at my annual physical in December that my vitamin D levels were low. Knowing what I know now, it was easy to see why I wasn't going back into remission.

As I began to rectify these issues, slowly my psoriasis began to heal again. I gradually reduced my sugar intake and went back to avoiding gluten. I returned to my usual 1-4 alcoholic drinks per month. I worked diligently on reducing my stress levels by meditating more, practicing gratitude, and engaging in stimulating yet relaxing activities like doing jigsaw puzzles, crossword puzzles, and reading for pleasure. I started taking 1,000 IUs of vitamin D per day, as recommended by my doctor. My psoriasis began to heal. Finally, six months later in March 2021, I went back into remission.

This experience has cemented my belief that we need to expand our understanding of healing in the medical community, and look towards healing matrices that take into consideration multifactorial elements like food, environment, the microbiome, genetics, and lifestyle instead of single quick fixes. It's no longer appropriate to try and pinpoint one single cause for chronic diseases – we must be smarter than that. It's time we seriously reckon with how this modern world that we have created around us is negatively impacting our health. There is much work to be done in improving the medical community, but if I can help other psoriasis sufferers by sharing my knowledge and experience, then that is progress in the right direction. I sincerely hope from the bottom of my heart that your psoriasis journey will be as full of healing and increased self-awareness as mine has been – you deserve it!

Appendix: Resources

Candida Screening Form

Take this comprehensive questionnaire to obtain a better idea if your health problems are related to *Candida albicans* or not. Questions in Section A focus on your medical history, including factors that promote the growth of *Candida albicans* and that frequently are found in people with *Candida*-related health problems. In Section B, you will find a list of main symptoms that are often present in people with excessive *Candida*, while Section C consists of other symptoms that are sometimes seen.

Section A: Medical History

Circle or highlight the points on the right if you answer "yes" to the question.

1. Have you taken an antibiotic for 1 month or longer?	35
2. Have you at any time in your life taken broad spectrum antibiotics or other antibacterial medication for 2 months or longer, or in shorter courses 4 or more times in a 1 year period?	35
3. Have you ever taken a broad spectrum antibiotic drug?	6
4. Have you, at any time in your life, been bothered by persistent prostatitis, vaginitis or other problems affecting your reproductive organs?	25
5. Are you bothered by memory or concentration problems – do you sometimes feel spaced out or mentally foggy?	20
6. Do you ever feel "sick all over"?	20
7. <u>People assigned female only</u>: Have you been pregnant... ...2 or more times? ...1 time?	5 3
8. <u>People assigned female only</u>: Have you taken birth control pills... ...for more than 2 years? ...for 6 months to 2 years?	15 8
9. Have you taken steroids orally, by injection, or inhalation? For more than 2 weeks? For 2 weeks or less?	15 6
10. Does exposure to perfumes, laundromat odors, or other chemicals provoke... ...moderate to severe irritation or other symptoms? ...mild irritation or other symptoms?	20 5
11. Does tobacco smoke really bother you?	10
12. Are your symptoms worse on damp, muggy days or in moldy places?	20
13. Have you had athlete's foot, ringworm, "jock itch", or other chronic fungal infections of the skin or nails? Have such infections been... ...severe or persistent? ...mild to moderate?	20 10
14. Do you crave sugar, sweets, or products containing potato, corn, or wheat?	10
TOTAL SCORE, Section A → → →	

Section B: Major Symptoms

For each of your symptoms, write the corresponding number to the right:

If a symptom is occasional or mild..............................3 points
If a symptom is frequent and/or moderately severe.....6 points
If a symptom is severe and/or disabling ....9 points

Add the total score and record it at the end of section B.

1. Fatigue or lethargy	
2. Feeling "drained"	
3. Depression or manic depression	
4. Numbness, burning, or tingling	
5. Headache	
6. Muscle aches	
7. Muscle weakness or paralysis	
8. Pain and/or swelling in joints	
9. Abdominal pain	
10. Constipation and/or diarrhea	
11. Bloating, intestinal gas, or irritate bowel syndrome (IBS) diagnosis	
12. People assigned female only: Troublesome vaginal burning, itching, or discharge	
13. People assigned male only: Prostatitis	
14. People assigned male only: Impotence, erectile dysfunction	
15. Loss of sexual desire or feeling	
16. Endometriosis or infertility	
17. People assigned female only: Cramps and/or other menstrual irregularities	
18. People assigned female only: Severe PMS and/or painful periods	
19. High anxiety or chronic stress	
20. Cold hands or feet, low body temperature	
21. Hypothyroidism	
22. Shaking or irritable when hungry, being "hangry"	
23. Urinary tract infections, bladder infections, and/or vaginal yeast infections	
TOTAL SCORE, Section B → → →	

Section C: Other Symptoms

For each of your symptoms, write the corresponding number to the right:

If a symptom is occasional or mild .... 1 point

If a symptom is frequent and/or moderately severe .....2 points

If a symptom is severe and/or disabling.......................3 points

Add the total score and record it at the end of this section.

1. Drowsiness, including inappropriate drowsiness	
2. Irritability	
3. Incoordination	
4. Frequent mood swings	
5. Insomnia	
6. Dizziness/loss of balance	
7. Pressure above ears, feeling of head swelling	
8. Sinus problems, constantly clearing throat, and/or poor sense of smell	
9. Tendency to bruise easily	
10. Eczema or acne	
11. Psoriasis	
12. Chronic hives (urticaria)	
13. Indigestion or heartburn	
14. Sensitivity to milk, wheat, corn, or other common foods	
15. Mucus in stools	
16. Rectal itching, hemorrhoids	
17. Dry mouth or throat	
18. Thrush or mouth rashes, including "white" tongue	
19. Bad breath	
20. Foot, hair, or body odor not relieved by washing	
21. Nasal congestion and/or post-nasal drip	
22. Nasal itching	
23. Sore throat	
24. Laryngitis, loss of voice	
25. Cough or recurrent bronchitis	
26. Pain or tightness in chest	
27. Wheezing or shortness of breath	
28. Urinary frequency or urgency	
29. Burning on urination	
30. Spots in front of eyes or erratic vision	
31. Burning or tearing eyes	
32. Recurrent infections or fluid in ears	
33. Ear pain or deafness	
TOTAL SCORE, Section C → → →	

Now, add up all the total scores for a grand total:

TOTAL SCORE, Section A → → →	
TOTAL SCORE, Section B → → →	
TOTAL SCORE, Section C → → →	
GRAND TOTAL:	

REVIEW YOUR RESULTS:

For people assigned female, yeast-connected health problems are:
- Almost certainly present with a grand total >180
- Probably present with a grand total >120
- Possibly present with a grand total with >60

For people assigned male, yeast-connected health problems are:
- Almost certainly present with a grand total >140
- Probably present with a grand total >90
- Possibly present with a grand total with >40

Please note: Scores in people assigned female will run higher, as several items in the questionnaire apply exclusively to them while only two apply exclusively to people assigned male.[1]

Eating Attitudes Test (EAT)

The Eating Attitudes Test (EAT-26) is a widely used and accepted standardized screening form to measure common symptoms and characteristics of eating disorders. This test cannot definitively diagnose an eating disorder and does not take the place of a professional consultation, but those who score 20 or higher should seek further medical attention from a qualified provider such as a therapist, primary care doctor, psychiatrist, or other mental health provider with experience treating eating disorders. However, a low score does not mean that you should not seek help if you are concerned.

Fill out the form below as accurately, honestly and completely as possible. There are no right or wrong answers.

Section A:

1. Birthdate: _____

2. Gender: _____

3. Height (in feet and inches): _____

4. Current Weight (in pounds):_____

5. Highest Weight (excluding pregnancy): _____

6. Lowest Adult Weight:_____

7. Ideal Weight: _____

Section B:

Please circle a response for each of the following statements:

Statements:	Always	Usually	Often	Sometimes	Rarely	Never
I am terrified about being overweight.	3	2	1	0	0	0
I avoid eating when I am hungry.	3	2	1	0	0	0
I find myself preoccupied with food.	3	2	1	0	0	0
I have gone on eating binges where I feel that I may not be able to stop.	3	2	1	0	0	0
I cut my food into small pieces.	3	2	1	0	0	0
I am aware of the calorie content of foods that I eat.	3	2	1	0	0	0
I particularly avoid food with a high carbohydrate content (i.e., bread, rice, potatoes, etc.)	3	2	1	0	0	0
I feel that others would prefer it if I ate more.	3	2	1	0	0	0
I vomit after I have eaten.	3	2	1	0	0	0
I feel extremely guilty after eating.	3	2	1	0	0	0
I am preoccupied with a desire to be thinner.	3	2	1	0	0	0
I think about burning up calories when I exercise.	3	2	1	0	0	0
Other people think that I am too thin.	3	2	1	0	0	0
I am preoccupied with the thought of having fat on my body.	3	2	1	0	0	0
I take longer than others to eat my meals.	3	2	1	0	0	0
I avoid foods with sugar in them.	3	2	1	0	0	0
I eat diet foods.	3	2	1	0	0	0
I feel that food controls my life.	3	2	1	0	0	0
I display self-control around food.	3	2	1	0	0	0
I feel that others pressure me to eat.	3	2	1	0	0	0
I give too much time and thought to food.	3	2	1	0	0	0
I feel uncomfortable after eating sweets.	3	2	1	0	0	0
I engage in dieting behavior.	3	2	1	0	0	0
I like my stomach to be empty.	3	2	1	0	0	0
I have the impulse to vomit after meals.	3	2	1	0	0	0
I enjoy trying new rich foods.	0	0	0	1	2	3
Add up subtotal for each column:						

REVIEW YOUR RESULTS:

Once you have obtained the subtotals for each column, then add each subtotal together for the grand total. A score of 20 or higher indicates a "high level of concern about dieting, body weight, or problematic eating behaviors is present and warrants further investigation by a qualified professional." However, scores below 20 can still be consistent with eating disorders.

Section C:

Please mark a response for each of the following behaviors:

In the past 6 months have you:	Never	Once a month or less	2 - 3 times a month	Once a week	2 - 6 times a week	Once a day or more
Gone on eating binges where you feel that you may not be able to stop	1	2	3	4	5	6
Ever made yourself sick (vomited) to control your weight or shape	7	8	9	10	11	12
Ever used laxatives, diet pills or diuretics (water pills) to control your weight or shape	13	14	15	16	17	18
Exercised more than 60 minutes a day to lose or to control your weight	19	20	21	22	23	24
Lost 20 pounds or more in the past 6 months	25	☐ Yes			26	☐ No
Add up total for each column:						

Review Your Results:

See if you marked a response in any of the boxes numbered: 3, 4, 5, 6, 8, 9, 10, 11, 12, 14, 15, 16, 17, 18, 24, and 25. If so, then you should seek evaluation from a qualified provider such as a primary care doctor, psychiatrist, or other mental health provider with experience treating eating disorders.

If you marked boxes 1, 2, 7, 13, 19, 20, 21, 22, 23, and 26, then there is less likely a reason for concern. However, a full examination by a qualified medical professional may still be warranted.[2]

Calculate Psoriasis Area & Severity Index (PASI)

The Psoriasis Area and Severity Index (PASI) is a quantitative way to measure the
   severity of your psoriasis. It uses the amount of skin covered by psoriasis plus its appearance to generate a score. This can be tracked over time to help measure your improvements and healing process.

Instructions:

Part A
1. Identify the areas with psoriasis on your head, arms, torso, and legs.
2. For each of these areas, evaluate the redness, thickness, and scaling present on the skin. Use the psoriasis area score to indicate the severity of these characteristics in each bodily area. Write the corresponding number for the severity of each characteristic by body area in the corresponding empty box in Part A.
3. Sum the total of each area.

Part B
1. Identify what percentage of each body area is covered by psoriasis. Find the corresponding 1 - 6 score. Write the corresponding score by body area into each empty box in Part B.
2. Multiply the scores from each body area in Part A by the scores in Part B. Put the total in the Subtitles (C) row.
3. Multiply each total from Subtotals (C) by the corresponding Body Surface Area to find Totals (D).
4. Add together all values in Totals (D) to identify your PASI.

PART A:

Psoriasis Characteristic	Psoriasis Area Score	Head Score:	Arms Score:	Torso Score:	Legs Score:
Redness	0 = None				
Thickness	1 = Slight 2 = Moderate				
Scaling	3 = Severe 4 = Very severe				
Below, add together each column for each body region to give 4 separate totals (A):					
Psoriasis Area Score Total (A)					

PART B:

Percentage Area Affected	Area Score	Head Score:	Arms Score:	Torso Score:	Legs Score:
Indicate the percentage for each body region affected by psoriasis using the 1-6 scale	0 = 0% 1 = 1 - 9% 2 = 10 - 29% 3 = 30 - 49% 4 = 50 - 69% 5 = 70 - 89% 6 = 90 - 100%				
Multiply Psoriasis Area Score Total (A) by the above scores for each body region. This will provide 4 individual subtotals (C) below.					
Subtotals (C)					
Multiply each of the above Subtotals (C) by the numbers below, which represent the amount of body surface area represented by that region. (0.1 for head, 0.2 for arms, 0.3 for torso, and 0.4 for legs.)					
Body Surface Area		x 0.1	x 0.2	x 0.3	x 0.4
Totals (D)					
Add together all the scores in the Totals (D) row for your final score					
Final PASI Score: _____ [3]					

ENDNOTES

Introduction
1. "About Psoriasis" National Psoriasis Foundation, 14 January 2021, https://www.psoriasis.org/about-psoriasis/.
2. "How Common Is Psoriatic Arthritis in People with Psoriasis?" Arthritis Foundation, http://blog.arthritis.org/psoriatic-arthritis/psoriatic-arthritis-psoriasis/. Accessed May 6, 2020.
3. Cojocaru, M et al. "Multiple autoimmune syndrome." *Maedica* vol. 5,2 (2010): 132-4.
4. Vighi, G et al. "Allergy and the gastrointestinal system." *Clinical and experimental immunology* vol. 153 Suppl 1,Suppl 1 (2008): 3-6. doi:10.1111/j.1365-2249.2008.03713.x

The Game Plan
1. Raevuori, Anu et al. "The increased risk for autoimmune diseases in patients with eating disorders." *PloS one* vol. 9,8 e104845. 22 Aug. 2014, doi:10.1371/journal.pone.0104845
2. Hedman, Anna et al. "Bidirectional relationship between eating disorders and autoimmune diseases." *Journal of child psychology and psychiatry, and allied disciplines* vol. 60,7 (2019): 803-812. doi:10.1111/jcpp.12958
3. Jenco, Melissa. "Eating Disorders Linked to Immune System Diseases." *American Academy of Pediatrics*, 10 Nov. 2017, www.aappublications.org/news/2017/11/10/EatingDisorders111017.
4. "Statistics for Journalists." *Beat Eating Disorders*, www.beateatingdisorders.org.uk/media-centre/eating-disorder-statistics.
5. "Eating Disorder Facts & Statistics." *Eating Recovery Center*, www.eatingrecoverycenter.com/conditions/eating-disorders/facts-statistics.
6. "Eating Disorder Statistics: General & Diversity Stats." *National Association of Anorexia Nervosa and Associated Disorders*, anad.org/get-informed/about-eating-disorders/eating-disorders-statistics/.

7. Ekern, MS, LPC, Jacquelyn. "Eating Disorders: Symptoms, Signs, Causes & Articles For Treatment Help." *Eating Disorder Hope*, 11 July 2018, www.eatingdisorderhope.com/information/eating-disorder.

8. Denny, Kara N et al. "Intuitive eating in young adults. Who is doing it, and how is it related to disordered eating behaviors?." *Appetite* vol. 60,1 (2013): 13-19. doi:10.1016/j.appet.2012.09.029

9. "Psoriasis: More than Skin Deep." Harvard Health, Harvard Medical School, 20 June 2019, www.health.harvard.edu/diseases-and-conditions/psoriasis-more-than-skin-deep.

10. "Life with Psoriasis." *National Psoriasis Foundation*, 2 Nov. 2020, www.psoriasis.org/life-with-psoriasis/.

11. Tribole, Evelyn, and Elyse Resch. *Intuitive Eating: A Revolutionary Anti-Diet Approach.* 4th ed., St. Martin's Essentials, 2020.

12. "The Health at Every Size® (HAES®) Approach." *ASDAH*, The Association for Size Diversity and Health (ASDAH), asdah.org/health-at-every-size-haes-approach/.

13. Vighi, G et al. "Allergy and the gastrointestinal system." *Clinical and experimental immunology* vol. 153 Suppl 1,Suppl 1 (2008): 3-6. doi:10.1111/j.1365-2249.2008.03713.x

14. "Can Genes Be Turned on and off in Cells?" *MedlinePlus*, U.S. National Library of Medicine, 18 Sept. 2020, medlineplus.gov/genetics/understanding/howgeneswork/geneonoff/.

The 10 Principles of Intuitive Eating
1. Tribole, Evelyn, and Elyse Resch. *Intuitive Eating: A Revolutionary Anti-Diet Approach.* 4th ed., St. Martin's Essentials, 2020.

Strategy #1: Foods & Nutrients to Eat More Of!
1. Barrea, L., Balato, N., Di Somma, C. *et al.* Nutrition and psoriasis: is there any association between the severity of the disease and adherence to the Mediterranean diet?. *J Transl Med* 13, 18 (2015). https://doi.org/10.1186/s12967-014-0372-1

2. Afifi, Ladan et al. "Dietary Behaviors in Psoriasis: Patient-Reported Outcomes from a U.S. National Survey." *Dermatology and therapy* vol. 7,2 (2017): 227-242. doi:10.1007/s13555-017-0183-4

3. Yildirim, M et al. "The role of oxidants and antioxidants in psoriasis." *Journal of the European Academy of Dermatology and Venereology : JEADV* vol. 17,1 (2003): 34-6. doi:10.1046/j.1468-3083.2003.00641.

4. Prussick, Ronald et al. "Psoriasis Improvement in Patients Using Glutathione-enhancing, Nondenatured Whey Protein Isolate: A Pilot Study." *The Journal of clinical and aesthetic dermatology* vol. 6,10 (2013): 23-6.

5 ."Psoriasis: More than Skin Deep." Harvard Health, Harvard Medical School, 20 June 2019, www.health.harvard.edu/diseases-and-conditions/psoriasis-more-than-skin-deep.

6 "Life with Psoriasis." *National Psoriasis Foundation*, 2 Nov. 2020, www.psoriasis.org/life-with-psoriasis/.

7. Trafford AM, Parisi R, Kontopantelis E, Griffiths CEM, Ashcroft DM. Association of Psoriasis With the Risk of Developing or Dying of Cancer: A Systematic Review and Meta-analysis. *JAMA Dermatol.* 2019;155(12):1390–1403. doi:10.1001/jamadermatol.2019.3056

8. Galland, Leo. "Diet and inflammation." *Nutrition in clinical practice : official publication of the American Society for Parenteral and Enteral Nutrition* vol. 25,6 (2010): 634-40. doi:10.1177/0884533610385703

9. Woo, Vivienne, and Theresa Alenghat. "Host-microbiota interactions: epigenomic regulation." *Current opinion in immunology* vol. 44 (2017): 52-60. doi:10.1016/j.coi.2016.12.001

10. Caminero, A., Meisel, M., Jabri, B. *et al.* Mechanisms by which gut microorganisms influence food sensitivities. *Nat Rev Gastroenterol Hepatol* 16, 7–18 (2019). https://doi.org/10.1038/s41575-018-0064-z

11. Minihane, Anne M et al. "Low-grade inflammation, diet composition and health: current research evidence and its translation." *The British journal of nutrition* vol. 114,7 (2015): 999-1012. doi:10.1017/S0007114515002093

12. Anwar, H et al. (2019). Gut Microbiome: A New Organ System in Body. *Eukaryotic Microbiology.* 10.5772/intechopen.89634.

13. Baquero, F, and C Nombela. "The microbiome as a human organ." *Clinical microbiology and infection : the official publication of the European Society of Clinical Microbiology and Infectious Diseases* vol. 18 Suppl 4 (2012): 2-4. doi:10.1111/j.1469-0691.2012.03916.x

14. Westreich, Sam. "What Is a Microbiome - a Scientist's Explanation of How Our Newest Organ Affects Us." *Medium*, 31 July 2018, medium.com/@westwise/what-is-a-microbiome-a-scientists-explanation-of-how-our-newest-organ-affects-us-ac04c22d4b49.

15. Barrea, L., Balato, N., Di Somma, C. *et al.* Nutrition and psoriasis: is there any association between the severity of the disease and adherence to the Mediterranean diet?. *J Transl Med* 13, 18 (2015). https://doi.org/10.1186/s12967-014-0372-1

16. Afifi, Ladan et al. "Dietary Behaviors in Psoriasis: Patient-Reported Outcomes from a U.S. National Survey." *Dermatology and therapy* vol. 7,2 (2017): 227-242. doi:10.1007/s13555-017-0183-4

17. Barrea, L., Macchia, P.E., Tarantino, G. *et al.* Nutrition: a key environmental dietary factor in clinical severity and cardio-metabolic risk in psoriatic male patients evaluated by 7-day food-frequency

questionnaire. *J Transl Med* 13, 303 (2015).
https://doi.org/10.1186/s12967-015-0658-y

18. "Should You Be Taking an Omega-3 Supplement?" *Harvard Health Publishing*, Harvard Medical School, Apr. 2019,
www.health.harvard.edu/staying-healthy/should-you-be-taking-an-omega-3-supplement.

19. "Omega-3 Fatty Acids." *Office of Dietary Supplements*, National Institute of Health, 17 Oct. 2019,
ods.od.nih.gov/factsheets/Omega3FattyAcids-HealthProfessional/.

20. Daley, Cynthia A et al. "A review of fatty acid profiles and antioxidant content in grass-fed and grain-fed beef." *Nutrition journal* vol. 9 10. 10 Mar. 2010, doi:10.1186/1475-2891-9-10

21. "Research Shows Eggs from Pastured Chickens May Be More Nutritious." *Penn State News*, Penn State University, 20 July 2010, news.psu.edu/story/166143/2010/07/20/research-shows-eggs-pastured-chickens-may-be-more-nutritious.

22. Walls-Thumma, Dawn. "What Are the Nutritional Differences Between Pasture-Fed Chickens Vs. Non?" *Home Guides | SF Gate*, 21 Nov. 2017, homeguides.sfgate.com/nutritional-differences-between-pasturefed-chickens-vs-non-79222.html

23 Pahwa R, Goyal A, Bansal P, et al. Chronic Inflammation. [Updated 2020 Mar 2]. In: StatPearls [Internet]. Treasure Island (FL): StatPearls Publishing; 2020 Jan-. Available from:
https://www.ncbi.nlm.nih.gov/books/NBK493173/

24. Millsop, Jillian W et al. "Diet and psoriasis, part III: role of nutritional supplements." *Journal of the American Academy of Dermatology* vol. 71,3 (2014): 561-9. doi:10.1016/j.jaad.2014.03.016

25. Madden, Seonad K et al. "How lifestyle factors and their associated pathogenetic mechanisms impact psoriasis." *Clinical nutrition (Edinburgh, Scotland)* vol. 39,4 (2020): 1026-1040.
doi:10.1016/j.clnu.2019.05.006

26. Jindal, Shanu, and Nitin Jindal. "Psoriasis and Cardiovascular Diseases: A Literature Review to Determine the Causal Relationship." *Cureus* vol. 10,2 e2195. 15 Feb. 2018, doi:10.7759/cureus.2195

27. Jain, A P et al. "Omega-3 fatty acids and cardiovascular disease." *European review for medical and pharmacological sciences* vol. 19,3 (2015): 441-5.

28. Rajaei, Elham et al. "The Effect of Omega-3 Fatty Acids in Patients With Active Rheumatoid Arthritis Receiving DMARDs Therapy: Double-Blind Randomized Controlled Trial." *Global journal of health science* vol. 8,7 18-25. 3 Nov. 2015, doi:10.5539/gjhs.v8n7p18

29. Neale, Elizabeth, et al. "Will Eating Nuts Make You Gain Weight?" *ScienceAlert*, 18 Feb. 2019, www.sciencealert.com/will-eating-nuts-make-you-gain-weight.
30. "Vitamin D: Fact Sheet for Health Professionals." *NIH Office of Dietary Supplements*, U.S. Department of Health and Human Services, 9 Oct. 2020, ods.od.nih.gov/factsheets/VitaminD-HealthProfessional/.
31. Aranow, Cynthia. "Vitamin D and the immune system." *Journal of investigative medicine : the official publication of the American Federation for Clinical Research* vol. 59,6 (2011): 881-6. doi:10.2310/JIM.0b013e31821b8755
32. "6 Things You Should Know about Vitamin D." *Harvard Health Publishing*, Harvard Medical School, 30 Oct. 2020, www.health.harvard.edu/staying-healthy/6-things-you-should-know-about-vitamin-d.
33. Gutierrez, Emilio et al. "Psoriasis: Latitude does make a difference." *Journal of the American Academy of Dermatology* vol. 77,2 (2017): e57. doi:10.1016/j.jaad.2017.03.049
34. Cantorna, Margherita T. "Why Getting Enough Vitamin D in Wintertime Is so Important." *The Washington Post*, 19 Jan. 2020, www.washingtonpost.com/health/why-getting-enough-vitamin-d-in-wintertime-is-so-important/2020/01/17/c3598082-3875-11ea-9541-9107303481a4_story.html.
35. Arango MT, Shoenfeld Y, Cervera R, et al. Infection and autoimmune diseases. In: Anaya JM, Shoenfeld Y, Rojas-Villarraga A, et al., editors. Autoimmunity: From Bench to Bedside [Internet]. Bogota (Colombia): El Rosario University Press; 2013 Jul 18. Chapter 19. Available from: https://www.ncbi.nlm.nih.gov/books/NBK459437/
36. Barrea, L., Savanelli, M.C., Di Somma, C. *et al.* Vitamin D and its role in psoriasis: An overview of the dermatologist and nutritionist. *Rev Endocr Metab Disord* 18, 195–205 (2017). https://doi.org/10.1007/s11154-017-9411-6
37. Altieri, B., Muscogiuri, G., Barrea, L. *et al.* Does vitamin D play a role in autoimmune endocrine disorders? A proof of concept. *Rev Endocr Metab Disord* 18, 335–346 (2017). https://doi.org/10.1007/s11154-016-9405-9
38. Wareeporn Disphanurat, Wongsiya Viarasilpa, Panlop Chakkavittumrong, Padcha Pongcharoen, "The Clinical Effect of Oral Vitamin D2 Supplementation on Psoriasis: A Double-Blind, Randomized, Placebo-Controlled Study", *Dermatology Research and Practice*, vol. 2019, Article ID 5237642, 9 pages, 2019. https://doi.org/10.1155/2019/5237642

39. "Healing Psoriasis From The Inside Out with Dr. Todd LePine." *The Doctor's Farmacy: House Call*, Dr. Mark Hyman, drhyman.com/blog/2020/10/16/podcast-hc27/.

40. Groeger, David et al. "Bifidobacterium infantis 35624 modulates host inflammatory processes beyond the gut." *Gut microbes* vol. 4,4 (2013): 325-39. doi:10.4161/gmic.25487

41. Metikurke Vijayashankar, Nithya Raghunath: Pustular psoriasis responding to Probiotics – a new insight. Our Dermatol Online. 2012; 3(4): 326-328

42. Codoñer, F.M., Ramírez-Bosca, A., Climent, E. *et al.* Gut microbial composition in patients with psoriasis. *Sci Rep* 8, 3812 (2018). https://doi.org/10.1038/s41598-018-22125-y

43. Campos, Marcelo. "Leaky Gut: What Is It, and What Does It Mean for You?" *Harvard Health Blog*, Harvard Medical School, 22 Oct. 2019, www.health.harvard.edu/blog/leaky-gut-what-is-it-and-what-does-it-mean-for-you-2017092212451.

44. Martínez-Augustin, Olga et al. "Food derived bioactive peptides and intestinal barrier function." *International journal of molecular sciences* vol. 15,12 22857-73. 9 Dec. 2014, doi:10.3390/ijms151222857

45. Humbert, P et al. "Intestinal permeability in patients with psoriasis." *Journal of dermatological science* vol. 2,4 (1991): 324-6. doi:10.1016/0923-1811(91)90057-5

46. Fasano, Alessio. "Zonulin, regulation of tight junctions, and autoimmune diseases." *Annals of the New York Academy of Sciences* vol. 1258,1 (2012): 25-33. doi:10.1111/j.1749-6632.2012.06538.

47. Basmaciyan, Louise et al. ""Candida Albicans Interactions With The Host: Crossing The Intestinal Epithelial Barrier"." *Tissue barriers* vol. 7,2 (2019): 1612661. doi:10.1080/21688370.2019.1612661

48. Cui, Y et al."Intestinal Barrier Function–Non-alcoholic Fatty Liver Disease Interactions and Possible Role of Gut Microbiota." *Journal of Agricultural and Food Chemistry* 2019 67 (10), 2754-2762. DOI: 10.1021/acs.jafc.9b00080.

49. Prussick, Ronald et al. "Nonalcoholic Fatty liver disease and psoriasis: what a dermatologist needs to know." *The Journal of clinical and aesthetic dermatology* vol. 8,3 (2015): 43-5.

50. "Patient Education: Increasing Fiber Intake." *UCSF Health* , University of California San Francisco, www.ucsfhealth.org/education/increasing-fiber-intake.

51. Damiani G, Bragazzi NL, McCormick TS, Pigatto PDM, Leone S, Pacifico A, Tiodorovic D, Di Franco S, Alfieri A, Fiore M. Gut microbiota and nutrient interactions with skin in psoriasis: A comprehensive review of animal and human studies. *World J Clin Cases* 2020; 8(6): 1002-1012

52. Ma, Yunsheng et al. "Association between dietary fiber and serum C-reactive protein." *The American journal of clinical nutrition* vol. 83,4 (2006): 760-6. doi:10.1093/ajcn/83.4.760

53. Raman, Ryan. "12 Foods That Contain Natural Digestive Enzymes." *Healthline*, 15 May 2018, www.healthline.com/nutrition/natural-digestive-enzymes.

54. Van Spaendonk, Hanne et al. "Regulation of intestinal permeability: The role of proteases." *World journal of gastroenterology* vol. 23,12 (2017): 2106-2123. doi:10.3748/wjg.v23.i12.2106

55. Viswanatha Swamy, A H M, and P A Patil. "Effect of some clinically used proteolytic enzymes on inflammation in rats." *Indian journal of pharmaceutical sciences* vol. 70,1 (2008): 114-7. doi:10.4103/0250-474X.40347

56. Lodish H, Berk A, Zipursky SL, et al. Molecular Cell Biology. 4th edition. New York: W. H. Freeman; 2000. Section 22.3, Collagen: The Fibrous Proteins of the Matrix. Available from: https://www.ncbi.nlm.nih.gov/books/NBK21582/

57. Koivukangas, V et al. "Increased collagen synthesis in psoriasis in vivo." *Archives of dermatological research* vol. 287,2 (1995): 171-5. doi:10.1007/BF01262327

58. Song, Wenkui et al. "Identification and Structure-Activity Relationship of Intestinal Epithelial Barrier Function Protective Collagen Peptides from Alaska Pollock Skin." *Marine drugs* vol. 17,8 450. 31 Jul. 2019, doi:10.3390/md17080450

59. Chen, Qianru et al. "Collagen peptides ameliorate intestinal epithelial barrier dysfunction in immunostimulatory Caco-2 cell monolayers via enhancing tight junctions." *Food & function* vol. 8,3 (2017): 1144-1151. doi:10.1039/c6fo01347c

60. Tinsley, Grant. "Glutamine: Benefits, Uses and Side Effects." *Healthline*, 13 Jan. 2018, www.healthline.com/nutrition/glutamine.

61. Murakami, Hitoshi et al. "Combination of BCAAs and glutamine enhances dermal collagen protein synthesis in protein-malnourished rats." *Amino acids* vol. 44,3 (2013): 969-76. doi:10.1007/s00726-012-1426-4

62. Armstrong, April W et al. "Metabolomics in psoriatic disease: pilot study reveals metabolite differences in psoriasis and psoriatic arthritis." *F1000Research* vol. 3 248. 21 Oct. 2014, doi:10.12688/f1000research.4709.1

63. Achamrah, Najate et al. "Glutamine and the regulation of intestinal permeability: from bench to bedside." *Current opinion in clinical nutrition and metabolic care* vol. 20,1 (2017): 86-91. doi:10.1097/MCO.0000000000000339

64. Dosychev, E A, and V N Bystrova. "Lechenie psoriaza preparatami griba "Chaga"" [Treatment of psoriasis using "Chaga" fungus preparations]. *Vestnik dermatologii i venerologii* vol. 47,5 (1973): 79-83.
65. Kim, Yeon-Ran. "Immunomodulatory Activity of the Water Extract from Medicinal Mushroom Inonotus obliquus." *Mycobiology* vol. 33,3 (2005): 158-62. doi:10.4489/MYCO.2005.33.3.158
66. Kim, Gi-Young et al. "Oral administration of proteoglycan isolated from Phellinus linteus in the prevention and treatment of collagen-induced arthritis in mice." *Biological & pharmaceutical bulletin* vol. 26,6 (2003): 823-31. doi:10.1248/bpb.26.823
67. Lull, Cristina et al. "Antiinflammatory and immunomodulating properties of fungal metabolites." *Mediators of inflammation* vol. 2005,2 (2005): 63-80. doi:10.1155/MI.2005.63
68. Reinagel, Monica. "What Are the Benefits of Drinking Aloe Juice?" *Scientific American*, 8 Dec. 2018, www.scientificamerican.com/article/what-are-the-benefits-of-drinking-aloe-juice/.
69. Gardner, Stephanie S. "The Link Between Psoriasis and Digestive Problems, IBD & Celiac Disease." *WebMD*, 24 Jan. 2019, www.webmd.com/skin-problems-and-treatments/psoriasis/psoriasis-digestive-disorders.
70. Mayo Clinic Staff. "Psoriasis: Diagnosis and Treatment." *Mayo Clinic*, Mayo Foundation for Medical Education and Research, 2 May 2020, www.mayoclinic.org/diseases-conditions/psoriasis/diagnosis-treatment/drc-20355845.
71. "Ulcerative Colitis." *Diseases and Conditions: Ulcerative Colitis*, NCH Healthcare System, 13 Oct. 2020, www.nchmd.org/education/mayo-health-library/details/CON-20312397.
72. Langmead, L et al. "Randomized, double-blind, placebo-controlled trial of oral aloe vera gel for active ulcerative colitis." *Alimentary pharmacology & therapeutics* vol. 19,7 (2004): 739-47. doi:10.1111/j.1365-2036.2004.01902.x
73. Syed, T A et al. "Management of psoriasis with Aloe vera extract in a hydrophilic cream: a placebo-controlled, double-blind study." *Tropical medicine & international health : TM & IH* vol. 1,4 (1996): 505-9. doi:10.1046/j.1365-3156.1996.d01-91.x
74. Choonhakarn, C et al. "A prospective, randomized clinical trial comparing topical aloe vera with 0.1% triamcinolone acetonide in mild to moderate plaque psoriasis." *Journal of the European Academy of Dermatology and Venereology* : JEADV vol. 24,2 (2010): 168-72. doi:10.1111/j.1468-3083.2009.03377.x

Strategy #2: Meal Timing
1. Pot, Gerda K., et al. "Meal Irregularity and Cardiometabolic Consequences: Results from Observational and Intervention Studies." *Proceedings of the Nutrition Society*, vol. 75, no. 4, 2016, pp. 475–486., doi:10.1017/S0029665116000239.
2. Tahara, Y. et al. "Chronobiology and nutrition." *Neuroscience*. 2013 Dec 3;253:78-88. doi: 10.1016/j.neuroscience.2013.08.049.
3. Johnston, J.D. (2014), Physiological links between circadian rhythms, metabolism and nutrition. Exp Physiol, 99: 1133-1137. doi:10.1113/expphysiol.2014.078295
4. Remröd, Charlotta et al. "Subjective stress reactivity in psoriasis - a cross sectional study of associated psychological traits." *BMC dermatology* vol. 15 6. 2 May. 2015, doi:10.1186/s12895-015-0026-x
5. Gaston, L et al. "Psoriasis and stress: a prospective study." *Journal of the American Academy of Dermatology*. 1987 Jul;17(1):82-6.
6. Verhoeven, E W M et al. "Individual differences in the effect of daily stressors on psoriasis: a prospective study." *The British journal of dermatology* vol. 161,2 (2009): 295-9. doi:10.1111/j.1365-2133.2009.09194.x
7. Tribole, Evelyn, and Elyse Resch. *Intuitive Eating: A Revolutionary Anti-Diet Approach*. 4th ed., St. Martin's Essentials, 2020.
8. Medical Research Council. "How eating feeds into the body clock." ScienceDaily. ScienceDaily, 25 April 2019. <www.sciencedaily.com/releases/2019/04/190425143607.htm>.
9. Crosby, Priya et al. "Insulin/IGF-1 Drives PERIOD Synthesis to Entrain Circadian Rhythms with Feeding Time." *Cell* vol. 177,4 (2019): 896-909.e20. doi:10.1016/j.cell.2019.02.017
10. Ando, Noriko et al. "Circadian Gene Clock Regulates Psoriasis-Like Skin Inflammation in Mice." *The Journal of investigative dermatology* vol. 135,12 (2015): 3001-3008. doi:10.1038/jid.2015.316
11. Lyons, Alexis B et al. "Circadian Rhythm and the Skin: A Review of the Literature." *The Journal of clinical and aesthetic dermatology* vol. 12,9 (2019): 42-45.
12. Pietrangelo, Ann, and Kristeen Cherney. "The Effects of Low Blood Sugar on Your Body." *Healthine*, 15 Aug. 2018, www.healthline.com/health/low-blood-sugar-effects-on-body.
13. Wehrens, Sophie M T et al. "Meal Timing Regulates the Human Circadian System." *Current biology : CB* vol. 27,12 (2017): 1768-1775.e3. doi:10.1016/j.cub.2017.04.059
14. Naidoo, Uma. "Eating Well to Help Manage Anxiety: Your Questions Answered." *Harvard Health Blog*, Harvard Medical School, 14 Mar. 2018,

www.health.harvard.edu/blog/eating-well-to-help-manage-anxiety-your-questions-answered-2018031413460.

15. Lad, Vasant. *The Complete Book of Ayurvedic Home Remedies.* Piatkus, 2006.

16. Adawi, Mohammad et al. "The Impact of Intermittent Fasting (Ramadan Fasting) on Psoriatic Arthritis Disease Activity, Enthesitis, and Dactylitis: A Multicentre Study." *Nutrients* vol. 11,3 601. 12 Mar. 2019, doi:10.3390/nu11030601

17. Damiani, Giovanni et al. "The Impact of Ramadan Fasting on the Reduction of PASI Score, in Moderate-To-Severe Psoriatic Patients: A Real-Life Multicenter Study." *Nutrients* 2019, 11(2), 277; https://doi.org/10.3390/nu11020277

18. Glick, Danielle et al. "Autophagy: cellular and molecular mechanisms." *The Journal of pathology* vol. 221,1 (2010): 3-12. doi:10.1002/path.2697

19. "2017 Award and Grant Recipients." *American Skin Association*, www.americanskin.org/research/recipients2017.php.

Strategy #3: Individual Eating Pattern Recommendations – Food Sensitivities

1. Fasano, Alessio. "Zonulin, regulation of tight junctions, and autoimmune diseases." *Annals of the New York Academy of Sciences* vol. 1258,1 (2012): 25-33. doi:10.1111/j.1749-6632.2012.06538.

2. Kelso, John M. "Unproven Diagnostic Tests for Adverse Reactions to Foods." *The journal of allergy and clinical immunology.* In practice vol. 6,2 (2018): 362-365. doi:10.1016/j.jaip.2017.08.021

3. "Food Allergies and Food Intolerances." *Harvard Health*, Harvard Medical School, May 2011, www.health.harvard.edu/allergies/food-allergies-and-food-intolerances.

4. Patenaude, Jan. "Inflammation and Food Sensitivities - Successful Treatment Begins With Patient-Centered Care." *Today's Dietitian*, Nov. 2011, www.todaysdietitian.com/newarchives/110211p18.shtml.

5. "Life with Psoriasis." *National Psoriasis Foundation*, https://www.psoriasis.org/life-with-psoriasis/.

6. Raevuori, Anu et al. "The increased risk for autoimmune diseases in patients with eating disorders." *PloS one* vol. 9,8 e104845. 22 Aug. 2014, doi:10.1371/journal.pone.0104845

7. Hedman, Anna et al. "Bidirectional relationship between eating disorders and autoimmune diseases." *Journal of child psychology and psychiatry, and allied disciplines* vol. 60,7 (2019): 803-812. doi:10.1111/jcpp.12958

8. Jenco, Melissa. "Eating Disorders Linked to Immune System Diseases." *American Academy of Pediatrics*, 10 Nov. 2017, www.aappublications.org/news/2017/11/10/EatingDisorders111017.
9. "Eating Disorder Statistics: General & Diversity Stats." *National Association of Anorexia Nervosa and Associated Disorders*, anad.org/get-informed/about-eating-disorders/eating-disorders-statistics/.
10. "Eating Disorder Facts & Statistics." *Eating Recovery Center*, www.eatingrecoverycenter.com/conditions/eating-disorders/facts-statistics.
11. "Statistics for Journalists." *Beat Eating Disorders*, www.beateatingdisorders.org.uk/media-centre/eating-disorder-statistics.
12. Raman, Ryan. "How to Do an Elimination Diet and Why." *Healthline*, 2 July 2017, www.healthline.com/nutrition/elimination-diet.
13. Bardone-Cone, Anna M et al. "The inter-relationships between vegetarianism and eating disorders among females." *Journal of the Academy of Nutrition and Dietetics* vol. 112,8 (2012): 1247-52. doi:10.1016/j.jand.2012.05.007
14. Afifi, Ladan et al. "Dietary Behaviors in Psoriasis: Patient-Reported Outcomes from a U.S. National Survey." *Dermatology and therapy* vol. 7,2 (2017): 227-242. doi:10.1007/s13555-017-0183-4
15. Cronin, C C, and F Shanahan. "Why is celiac disease so common in Ireland?." *Perspectives in biology and medicine* vol. 44,3 (2001): 342-52. doi:10.1353/pbm.2001.0045
16. Ludvigsson, Jonas F et al. "Screening for celiac disease in the general population and in high-risk groups." *United European gastroenterology journal* vol. 3,2 (2015): 106-20. doi:10.1177/2050640614561668
17. Catassi, C et al. "Why is coeliac disease endemic in the people of the Sahara?." *Lancet (London, England)* vol. 354,9179 (1999): 647-8. doi:10.1016/s0140-6736(99)02609-4
18. Adams, Jefferson. "High Rates of Celiac Disease and Detection in Finland." *Celiac.com*, 31 July 2009, www.celiac.com/articles.html/high-rates-of-celiac-disease-and-detection-in-finland-r1479/
19. Volta, U et al. "High prevalence of celiac disease in Italian general population." *Digestive diseases and sciences* vol. 46,7 (2001): 1500-5. doi:10.1023/a:1010648122797
20. "Dietary Modifications." *National Psoriasis Foundation*, 10 Oct. 2020, https://www.psoriasis.org/dietary-modifications/
21. Kolchak, Nikolai A et al. "Prevalence of antigliadin IgA antibodies in psoriasis vulgaris and response of seropositive patients to a gluten-free

diet." *Journal of multidisciplinary healthcare* vol. 11 13-19. 27 Dec. 2017, doi:10.2147/JMDH.S122256

22. "What's the Deal With Nightshade Vegetables?" *Health Essentials from Cleveland Clinic*, Cleveland Clinic, 20 Sept. 2019, health.clevelandclinic.org/whats-the-deal-with-nightshade-vegetables/.

23. Hart, Jane. "Solanine Poisoning – How Does It Happen?" *MSU Extension*, Michigan State University, 4 Feb. 2014, www.canr.msu.edu/news/solanine_poisoning_how_does_it_happen.

24. "Health Concerns About Dairy." *Physicians Committee for Responsible Medicine*, www.pcrm.org/good-nutrition/nutrition-information/health-concerns-about-dairy.

25. Williams, Paul V. "The Epidemiology of Milk Allergy in US Children." *AAP News & Journals Gateway*, American Academy of Pediatrics, Oct. 2013, pediatrics.aappublications.org/content/132/Supplement_1/S17.2. DOI: https://doi.org/10.1542/peds.2013-2294Z

26. Herbert, Diana et al. "High-Fat Diet Exacerbates Early Psoriatic Skin Inflammation Independent of Obesity: Saturated Fatty Acids as Key Players." *The Journal of investigative dermatology* vol. 138,9 (2018): 1999-2009. doi:10.1016/j.jid.2018.03.1522

27. Kunz, Manfred et al. "Psoriasis: Obesity and Fatty Acids." *Frontiers in immunology* vol. 10 1807. 31 Jul. 2019, doi:10.3389/fimmu.2019.01807

28. Aslam, Hajara et al. "The effects of dairy and dairy derivatives on the gut microbiota: a systematic literature review." *Gut microbes* vol. 12,1 (2020): 1799533. doi:10.1080/19490976.2020.1799533

29. "Rethinking Restrictive Diets: Should We Be Eating More Dairy and Carbs?" *Goop*, goop.com/wellness/health/rethinking-restrictive-diets-eating-dairy-carbs/.

30. Hermenau, Gail. "Weekly Crop Update: Metal Contamination in Vegetables – Cadmium Is Becoming a Concern." *UD Cooperative Extension*, University of Delaware, 28 June 2019, sites.udel.edu/weeklycropupdate/?p=13637.

31. "Fiber and Irritable Bowel Syndrome." *UPMC HealthBeat*, 26 Mar. 2016, share.upmc.com/2016/03/irritable-bowel-syndrome-high-fiber-diet/.

32. Mayo Clinic Staff. "Nutrition and Healthy Eating: Diverticulitis Diet." *Mayo Clinic*, Mayo Foundation for Medical Education and Research, 11 Oct. 2019, www.mayoclinic.org/healthy-lifestyle/nutrition-and-healthy-eating/in-depth/diverticulitis-diet/art-20048499.

33. Yong, Wai Chung et al. "Association between Psoriasis and Helicobacter pylori Infection: A Systematic Review and Meta-analysis."

Indian journal of dermatology vol. 63,3 (2018): 193-200.
doi:10.4103/ijd.IJD_531_17
34. Healthwise Staff. "H. Pylori Bacterial Infection: Care Instructions."
MyHealth.Alberta.ca, Government of Alberta, 12 Aug. 2019,
myhealth.alberta.ca/Health/aftercareinformation/pages/conditions.aspx?
hwid=uh3180.
35. Figura, N et al. "Food allergy and Helicobacter pylori infection."
Italian journal of gastroenterology and hepatology vol. 31,3 (1999): 186-
91.
36. Ma, Zheng Fei et al. "Food Allergy and Helicobacter pylori Infection:
A Systematic Review." *Frontiers in microbiology* vol. 7 368. 23 Mar.
2016, doi:10.3389/fmicb.2016.00368

*Strategy #4: Universal Eating Pattern Recommendations – Foods to
Reduce*
1. Afifi, Ladan et al. "Dietary Behaviors in Psoriasis: Patient-Reported
Outcomes from a U.S. National Survey." *Dermatology and therapy* vol.
7,2 (2017): 227-242. doi:10.1007/s13555-017-0183-4
2. Fitzgerald, Jenny. "Can You Drink Alcohol If You Have Psoriasis?"
Medical News Today, 10 Oct. 2018,
www.medicalnewstoday.com/articles/314623.
3. Bishehsari, Faraz et al. "Alcohol and Gut-Derived Inflammation."
Alcohol research : current reviews vol. 38,2 (2017): 163-171.
4. Barrea, Luigi et al. "Nutrition: a key environmental dietary factor in
clinical severity and cardio-metabolic risk in psoriatic male patients
evaluated by 7-day food-frequency questionnaire." *Journal of
translational medicine* vol. 13 303. 16 Sep. 2015, doi:10.1186/s12967-
015-0658-y
5. Avena, Nicole M et al. "Evidence for sugar addiction: behavioral and
neurochemical effects of intermittent, excessive sugar intake."
Neuroscience and biobehavioral reviews vol. 32,1 (2008): 20-39.
doi:10.1016/j.neubiorev.2007.04.019
6. "How Much Is Too Much? The Growing Concern over Too Much
Added Sugar in Our Diets." *SugarScience.UCSF.edu*, University of
California San Francisco, sugarscience.ucsf.edu/the-growing-concern-
of-overconsumption.html.
7. Townsend, G et al. "Dietary sugar silences a colonization factor in a
mammalian gut symbiont" *Proceedings of the National Academy of
Sciences* Jan 2019, 116 (1) 233-238; DOI: 10.1073/pnas.1813780115
8. Caporuscio, Jessica. "Does Sugar Cause Inflammation?" *Medical
News Today*, 19 Sept. 2019,
www.medicalnewstoday.com/articles/326386.

9. Do, Moon Ho et al. "High-Glucose or -Fructose Diet Cause Changes of the Gut Microbiota and Metabolic Disorders in Mice without Body Weight Change." *Nutrients* vol. 10,6 761. 13 Jun. 2018, doi:10.3390/nu10060761

10. Rademaker, Marius et al. "Psoriasis and infection. A clinical practice narrative." *The Australasian journal of dermatology* vol. 60,2 (2019): 91-98. doi:10.1111/ajd.12895

11. Lamps, Laura W et al. "Fungal infections of the gastrointestinal tract in the immunocompromised host: an update." *Advances in anatomic pathology* vol. 21,4 (2014): 217-27. doi:10.1097/PAP.0000000000000016

12. Silver, Natalie. "Are Candida and Psoriasis Related?" *Healthline*, 23 Mar. 2018, www.healthline.com/health/psoriasis-and-candida#types-of-candida.

13. Taheri Sarvtin, Mehdi et al. "Evaluation of candidal colonization and specific humoral responses against Candida albicans in patients with psoriasis." *International journal of dermatology* vol. 53,12 (2014): e555-60. doi:10.1111/ijd.12562

14. Waldman, A et al. "Incidence of Candida in psoriasis—a study on the fungal flora of psoriatic patients." *Mycoses* vol. 44,3-4 (2001): 77-81. doi:10.1046/j.1439-0507.2001.00608.x

15. Moyes, David L et al. "Candidalysin is a fungal peptide toxin critical for mucosal infection." *Nature* vol. 532,7597 (2016): 64-8. doi:10.1038/nature17625

16. Bertling, Anne et al. "Candida albicans and its metabolite gliotoxin inhibit platelet function via interaction with thiols." *Thrombosis and haemostasis* vol. 104,2 (2010): 270-8. doi:10.1160/TH09-11-0769

17. "Alcohol Metabolism: An Update." *National Institute on Alcohol Abuse and Alcoholism*, U.S. Department of Health and Human Services, July 2007, pubs.niaaa.nih.gov/publications/aa72/aa72.htm.

18. Basmaciyan, Louise et al. ""Candida Albicans Interactions With The Host: Crossing The Intestinal Epithelial Barrier"." *Tissue barriers* vol. 7,2 (2019): 1612661. doi:10.1080/21688370.2019.1612661

19. Kumamoto, Carol A. "Inflammation and gastrointestinal Candida colonization." *Current opinion in microbiology* vol. 14,4 (2011): 386-91. doi:10.1016/j.mib.2011.07.015

20. Jason E. Hawkes, Bernice Y. Yan, Tom C. Chan, James G. Krueger. "Discovery of the IL-23/IL-17 Signaling Pathway and the Treatment of Psoriasis" *The Journal of Immunology* September 15, 2018, 201 (6) 1605-1613; DOI: 10.4049/jimmunol.1800013

21. Sissons, Beth. "How to Recognize Candida in Stool." *Medical News Today*, 16 Aug. 2019, www.medicalnewstoday.com/articles/326084.

22. Van Ende, Mieke et al. "Sugar Sensing and Signaling in *Candida albicans* and *Candida glabrata.*" *Frontiers in microbiology* vol. 10 99. 30 Jan. 2019, doi:10.3389/fmicb.2019.00099

23. Santos-Longhurst, Adrienne. "What a Candida Die-Off Is and Why It Makes You Feel So Lousy." *Healthline*, 28 June 2019, www.healthline.com/health/body/candida-die-off.

24. Villines, Zawn. "What to Know about Candida Die-Off." *Medical News Today* , 26 Feb. 2020, www.medicalnewstoday.com/articles/candida-die-off?c=202284531785.

25. Gunsalus, Kearney T W et al. "Manipulation of Host Diet To Reduce Gastrointestinal Colonization by the Opportunistic Pathogen Candida albicans." *mSphere* vol. 1,1 e00020-15. 18 Nov. 2015, doi:10.1128/mSphere.00020-15

26. Jensen, Thomas et al. "Fructose and sugar: A major mediator of non-alcoholic fatty liver disease." Journal of hepatology vol. 68,5 (2018): 1063-1075. doi:10.1016/j.jhep.2018.01.019

27. Prussick, Ronald et al. "Nonalcoholic Fatty liver disease and psoriasis: what a dermatologist needs to know." *The Journal of clinical and aesthetic dermatology* vol. 8,3 (2015): 43-5.

28. Holm, Jesper Grønlund, and Simon Francis Thomsen. "Type 2 diabetes and psoriasis: links and risks." *Psoriasis (Auckland, N.Z.)* vol. 9 1-6. 17 Jan. 2019, doi:10.2147/PTT.S159163

29. Jacques, Angela et al. "The impact of sugar consumption on stress driven, emotional and addictive behaviors." *Neuroscience and biobehavioral reviews* vol. 103 (2019): 178-199. doi:10.1016/j.neubiorev.2019.05.021

30. Abu-Darwish, M S et al. "Essential oil of common sage (Salvia officinalis L.) from Jordan: assessment of safety in mammalian cells and its antifungal and anti-inflammatory potential." *BioMed research international* vol. 2013 (2013): 538940. doi:10.1155/2013/538940

31. Chami, N et al. "Study of anticandidal activity of carvacrol and eugenol in vitro and in vivo." *Oral microbiology and immunology* vol. 20,2 (2005): 106-11. doi:10.1111/j.1399-302X.2004.00202.x

32. Tsutsumi-Arai, Chiaki et al. "Grapefruit seed extract effectively inhibits the Candida albicans biofilms development on polymethyl methacrylate denture-base resin." *PloS one* vol. 14,5 e0217496. 28 May. 2019, doi:10.1371/journal.pone.0217496

33. Hussain, Hidayat et al. "Lapachol: an overview." *Reviews and accounts* vol. 2007,2 , https://doi.org/10.3998/ark.5550190.0008.204

34. Rosenbloom, Cara. "What Is Ultra-Processed Food and How Can You Eat Less of It?" *Heart and Stroke Foundation of Canada*, www.heartandstroke.ca/articles/what-is-ultra-processed-food.

35. Laseter, Elizabeth. "What Is Ultra-Processed Food?" *Cooking Light*, 21 Feb. 2019, www.cookinglight.com/eating-smart/nutrition-101/what-is-ultra-processed-food.

36. Jaliman, Debra. "What You Should Know About Psoriasis and Your Diet." *WebMD*, 8 Nov. 2019, www.webmd.com/skin-problems-and-treatments/psoriasis/psoriasis-avoid-foods.

37. Lerner, A et al. "Changes in intestinal tight junction permeability associated with industrial food additives explain the rising incidence of autoimmune disease." *Autoimmunity Reviews*, Volume 14, Issue 6, 2015, Pages 479-489, ISSN 1568-9972, https://doi.org/10.1016/j.autrev.2015.01.009.

38. "NIH Study Finds Heavily Processed Foods Cause Overeating and Weight Gain." *National Institutes of Health*, U.S. Department of Health and Human Services, 16 May 2019, www.nih.gov/news-events/news-releases/nih-study-finds-heavily-processed-foods-cause-overeating-weight-gain.

39. Chen, Xiaojia et al. "Consumption of ultra-processed foods and health outcomes: a systematic review of epidemiological studies." *Nutrition journal* vol. 19,1 86. 20 Aug. 2020, doi:10.1186/s12937-020-00604-1

40. Delahunty, T et al. "Intestinal permeability changes in rodents: a possible mechanism for degraded carrageenan-induced colitis." *Food and chemical toxicology : an international journal published for the British Industrial Biological Research Association* vol. 25,2 (1987): 113-8. doi:10.1016/0278-6915(87)90143-8

41. "Psoriasis: More than Skin Deep." Harvard Health, Harvard Medical School, 20 June 2019, www.health.harvard.edu/diseases-and-conditions/psoriasis-more-than-skin-deep.

42. "Life with Psoriasis." *National Psoriasis Foundation*, https://www.psoriasis.org/life-with-psoriasis/.

43. Herbert, Diana et al. "High-Fat Diet Exacerbates Early Psoriatic Skin Inflammation Independent of Obesity: Saturated Fatty Acids as Key Players." *The Journal of investigative dermatology* vol. 138,9 (2018): 1999-2009. doi:10.1016/j.jid.2018.03.1522

44. Kunz, Manfred et al. "Psoriasis: Obesity and Fatty Acids." *Frontiers in immunology* vol. 10 1807. 31 Jul. 2019, doi:10.3389/fimmu.2019.01807

Strategy #5: Lifestyle Considerations
1. Tribole, Evelyn, and Elyse Resch. *Intuitive Eating: A Revolutionary Anti-Diet Approach.* 4th ed., St. Martin's Essentials, 2020.

2. "Stress Relievers: Tips to Tame Stress." *Mayo Clinic*, Mayo Foundation for Medical Education and Research, 12 Mar. 2019, www.mayoclinic.org/healthy-lifestyle/stress-management/in-depth/stress-relievers/art-20047257.
3. Park, Bum Jin et al. "The physiological effects of Shinrin-yoku (taking in the forest atmosphere or forest bathing): evidence from field experiments in 24 forests across Japan." *Environmental health and preventive medicine* vol. 15,1 (2010): 18-26. doi:10.1007/s12199-009-0086-9
4. Boyle, Neil Bernard et al. "The Effects of Magnesium Supplementation on Subjective Anxiety and Stress-A Systematic Review." *Nutrients* vol. 9,5 429. 26 Apr. 2017, doi:10.3390/nu9050429
5. DiNicolantonio, James J et al. "Subclinical magnesium deficiency: a principal driver of cardiovascular disease and a public health crisis." *Open heart* vol. 5,1 e000668. 13 Jan. 2018, doi:10.1136/openhrt-2017-000668
6. Panossian, Alexander, and Georg Wikman. "Effects of Adaptogens on the Central Nervous System and the Molecular Mechanisms Associated with Their Stress-Protective Activity." *Pharmaceuticals (Basel, Switzerland)* vol. 3,1 188-224. 19 Jan. 2010, doi:10.3390/ph3010188
7. Liao, Lian-Ying et al. "A preliminary review of studies on adaptogens: comparison of their bioactivity in TCM with that of ginseng-like herbs used worldwide." *Chinese medicine* vol. 13 57. 16 Nov. 2018, doi:10.1186/s13020-018-0214-9
8. Chandrasekhar, K et al. "A prospective, randomized double-blind, placebo-controlled study of safety and efficacy of a high-concentration full-spectrum extract of ashwagandha root in reducing stress and anxiety in adults." *Indian journal of psychological medicine* vol. 34,3 (2012): 255-62. doi:10.4103/0253-7176.106022
9. Wachtel-Galor S, Yuen J, Buswell JA, et al. Ganoderma lucidum (Lingzhi or Reishi): A Medicinal Mushroom. In: Benzie IFF, Wachtel-Galor S, editors. Herbal Medicine: Biomolecular and Clinical Aspects. 2nd edition. Boca Raton (FL): CRC Press/Taylor & Francis; 2011. Chapter 9. Available from: https://www.ncbi.nlm.nih.gov/books/NBK92757/
10. Remröd, Charlotta et al. "Subjective stress reactivity in psoriasis - a cross sectional study of associated psychological traits." *BMC dermatology* vol. 15 6. 2 May. 2015, doi:10.1186/s12895-015-0026-x
11. Gaston, L et al. "Psoriasis and stress: a prospective study." *Journal of the American Academy of Dermatology*. 1987 Jul;17(1):82-6.
12. Verhoeven, E W M et al. "Individual differences in the effect of daily stressors on psoriasis: a prospective study." *The British journal of*

dermatology vol. 161,2 (2009): 295-9. doi:10.1111/j.1365-2133.2009.09194.x

13. Blessing, Esther M et al. "Cannabidiol as a Potential Treatment for Anxiety Disorders." *Neurotherapeutics : the journal of the American Society for Experimental NeuroTherapeutics* vol. 12,4 (2015): 825-36. doi:10.1007/s13311-015-0387-1

14. Kaplan, Barbara L F et al. "The profile of immune modulation by cannabidiol (CBD) involves deregulation of nuclear factor of activated T cells (NFAT)." *Biochemical pharmacology* vol. 76,6 (2008): 726-37. doi:10.1016/j.bcp.2008.06.022

15. Prinz, J C. "The role of T cells in psoriasis." *Journal of the European Academy of Dermatology and Venereology : JEADV* vol. 17,3 (2003): 257-70. doi:10.1046/j.1468-3083.2003.00720.x

16. Wilkinson, Jonathan D, and Elizabeth M Williamson. "Cannabinoids inhibit human keratinocyte proliferation through a non-CB1/CB2 mechanism and have a potential therapeutic value in the treatment of psoriasis." *Journal of dermatological science* vol. 45,2 (2007): 87-92. doi:10.1016/j.jdermsci.2006.10.009

17. Jackson, Erica M. Ph.D., FACSM STRESS RELIEF, ACSM's Health & Fitness Journal: May/June 2013 - Volume 17 - Issue 3 - p 14-19 doi: 10.1249/FIT.0b013e31828cb1c9

18. Khoury, Bassam et al. "Mindfulness-based therapy: a comprehensive meta-analysis." *Clinical psychology review* vol. 33,6 (2013): 763-71. doi:10.1016/j.cpr.2013.05.005

19. Wium-Andersen, Marie Kim et al. "Elevated C-reactive protein levels, psychological distress, and depression in 73, 131 individuals." *JAMA psychiatry* vol. 70,2 (2013): 176-84. doi:10.1001/2013.jamapsychiatry.102

20. Risher, Brittany. "Chronic Illness Can Make It Hard to Trust Your Body." *The Paper Gown*, Zocdoc, 27 Sept. 2019, thepapergown.zocdoc.com/chronic-illness-can-make-it-hard-to-trust-your-body/.

21. Healthwise Staff. "Stress Management: Breathing Exercises for Relaxation." *Michigan Medicine*, University of Michigan , 15 Dec. 2019, www.uofmhealth.org/health-library/uz2255.

22. Bergland, Christopher. "Longer Exhalations Are an Easy Way to Hack Your Vagus Nerve." *Psychology Today*, 9 May 2019, www.psychologytoday.com/us/blog/the-athletes-way/201905/longer-exhalations-are-easy-way-hack-your-vagus-nerve.

23. "Meditation: In Depth." *National Center for Complementary and Integrative Health*, U.S. Department of Health and Human Services, Apr. 2016, www.nccih.nih.gov/health/meditation-in-depth.

24. Kabat-Zinn, J et al. "Influence of a mindfulness meditation-based stress reduction intervention on rates of skin clearing in patients with moderate to severe psoriasis undergoing phototherapy (UVB) and photochemotherapy (PUVA)." *Psychosomatic medicine* vol. 60,5 (1998): 625-32. doi:10.1097/00006842-199809000-00020
25. Lad, Vasant. *The Complete Book of Ayurvedic Home Remedies.* Piatkus, 2006.
26. Rumsey, Alissa. "7 Tips To Practice Intuitive Exercise: Intuitive Movement." *Alissa Rumsey Nutrition and Wellness*, 2 July 2019, alissarumsey.com/fitness/intuitive-exercise-tips/.
27. Nieman, David C. and Laurel M. Wentz. "The compelling link between physical activity and the body's defense system" Journal of Sport and Health Science, Volume 8, Issue 3, 2019, Pages 201-217, ISSN 2095-2546, https://doi.org/10.1016/j.jshs.2018.09.009. (http://www.sciencedirect.com/science/article/pii/S2095254618301005)
28. Sharif, Kassem et al. "Physical activity and autoimmune diseases: Get moving and manage the disease." *Autoimmunity reviews* vol. 17,1 (2018): 53-72. doi:10.1016/j.autrev.2017.11.010
29. "American Heart Association Recommendations for Physical Activity in Adults and Kids." *American Heart Association*, 18 Apr. 2018, www.heart.org/en/healthy-living/fitness/fitness-basics/aha-recs-for-physical-activity-in-adults.
30. Monda, Vincenzo et al. "Exercise Modifies the Gut Microbiota with Positive Health Effects." *Oxidative medicine and cellular longevity* vol. 2017 (2017): 3831972. doi:10.1155/2017/3831972
31. "Benefits of Exercise." *MedlinePlus*, U.S. National Library of Medicine, 20 Apr. 2020, medlineplus.gov/benefitsofexercise.html.
32. Drakaki, Eleni et al. "Air pollution and the skin." *Frontiers in environmental science* 2:11. doi: 10.3389/fenvs.2014.00011
33. Liaw, Fang-Yih et al. "Exploring the link between cadmium and psoriasis in a nationally representative sample." *Scientific reports* vol. 7,1 1723. 11 May. 2017, doi:10.1038/s41598-017-01827-9
34. Zhao, Chan-Na et al. "Emerging role of air pollution in autoimmune diseases." *Autoimmunity reviews* vol. 18,6 (2019): 607-614. doi:10.1016/j.autrev.2018.12.010
35. Gawda, Anna et al. "Air pollution, oxidative stress, and exacerbation of autoimmune diseases." *Central-European journal of immunology* vol. 42,3 (2017): 305-312. doi:10.5114/ceji.2017.70975
36. Faustini, Annunziata et al. "Short-term exposure to air pollution might exacerbate autoimmune diseases." *Environmental Epidemiology*: September 2018 - Volume 2 - Issue 3 - p e025 doi: 10.1097/EE9.0000000000000025

37. Press Release. "National Sleep Foundation Recommends New Sleep Times." *Sleep Foundation*, 2 Feb. 2015, www.sleepfoundation.org/press-release/national-sleep-foundation-recommends-new-sleep-times.

38. Suni, Eric. "What Is Sleep Hygiene?" *Sleep Foundation*, 14 Aug. 2020, www.sleepfoundation.org/sleep-hygiene.

39. Ger, Tzong-Yun et al. "Bidirectional Association Between Psoriasis and Obstructive Sleep Apnea: A Systematic Review and Meta-Analysis." *Scientific Reports* 10, 5931 (2020). https://doi.org/10.1038/s41598-020-62834-x

40. Skoie, I M et al. "Fatigue in psoriasis: a controlled study." *The British journal of dermatology* vol. 177,2 (2017): 505-512. doi:10.1111/bjd.15375

41. Melikoglu, Mehmet. "Sleep Quality and its Association with Disease Severity in Psoriasis." *The Eurasian journal of medicine* vol. 49,2 (2017): 124-127. doi:10.5152/eurasianjmed.2017.17132

42. Chiu, Hsien-Yi et al. "Concomitant Sleep Disorders Significantly Increase the Risk of Cardiovascular Disease in Patients with Psoriasis." *PloS one* vol. 11,1 e0146462. 8 Jan. 2016, doi:10.1371/journal.pone.0146462

43. Mubanga, Mwenya et al. "Dog ownership and the risk of cardiovascular disease and death - a nationwide cohort study." *Scientific reports* vol. 7,1 15821. 17 Nov. 2017, doi:10.1038/s41598-017-16118-6

44. Shiloh, Shoshana et al. "Reduction of state-anxiety by petting animals in a controlled laboratory experiment." *Anxiety, Stress & Coping*, 16:4, 387-395, DOI: 10.1080/1061580031000091582

45. Mubanga, Mwenya et al. "Dog ownership and the risk of cardiovascular disease and death - a nationwide cohort study." *Scientific reports* vol. 7,1 15821. 17 Nov. 2017, doi:10.1038/s41598-017-16118-6

46. Mayo Clinic Staff. "Exercise Helps Ease Arthritis Pain and Stiffness ." *Mayo Clinic*, Mayo Foundation for Medical Education and Research, 1 Dec. 2020, www.mayoclinic.org/diseases-conditions/arthritis/in-depth/arthritis/art-20047971.

47. Bridges, Alisha. "Should People With Psoriasis Have Pets?" *HealthCentral*, 31 Dec. 2019, www.healthcentral.com/article/psoriasis-and-health-advantages-of-owning-a-pet.

48. Atiya Rungjang, Jitlada Meephansan and Hok Bing Thio (June 2nd 2020). Skin and Gut Microbiota in Psoriasis: A Systematic Review [Online First], IntechOpen, DOI: 10.5772/intechopen.92686. Available from: https://www.intechopen.com/online-first/skin-and-gut-microbiota-in-psoriasis-a-systematic-review

49. Song, Se Jin et al. "Cohabiting family members share microbiota with one another and with their dogs." *eLife* vol. 2 e00458. 16 Apr. 2013, doi:10.7554/eLife.00458

Additional Thoughts

1. Murase, Jenny E et al. "Hormonal effect on psoriasis in pregnancy and post partum." *Archives of dermatology* vol. 141,5 (2005): 601-6. doi:10.1001/archderm.141.5.601
2. Damiani G, Bragazzi NL, McCormick TS, Pigatto PDM, Leone S, Pacifico A, Tiodorovic D, Di Franco S, Alfieri A, Fiore M. Gut microbiota and nutrient interactions with skin in psoriasis: A comprehensive review of animal and human studies. *World J Clin Cases* 2020; 8(6): 1002-1012
3. Waldman, A et al. "Incidence of Candida in psoriasis—a study on the fungal flora of psoriatic patients." *Mycoses* vol. 44,3-4 (2001): 77-81. doi:10.1046/j.1439-0507.2001.00608.x
4. Taheri Sarvtin, M., Shokohi, T., Hajheydari, Z., Yazdani, J. and Hedayati, M.T. (2014), Evaluation of candidal colonization and specific humoral responses against *Candida albicans* in patients with psoriasis. Int J Dermatol, 53: e555-e560. doi:10.1111/ijd.12562
5. Kim, Grace K, and James Q Del Rosso. "Drug-provoked psoriasis: is it drug induced or drug aggravated?: understanding pathophysiology and clinical relevance." *The Journal of clinical and aesthetic dermatology* vol. 3,1 (2010): 32-8.
6. Horton, Daniel B et al. "Antibiotic Exposure, Infection, and the Development of Pediatric Psoriasis: A Nested Case-Control Study." *JAMA dermatology* vol. 152,2 (2016): 191-9. doi:10.1001/jamadermatol.2015.3650
7. Saxena, V N, and Jaideep Dogra. "Long-term oral azithromycin in chronic plaque psoriasis: a controlled trial." *European journal of dermatology : EJD* vol. 20,3 (2010): 329-33. doi:10.1684/ejd.2010.0930
8. Saxena, V N, and J Dogra. "Long-term use of penicillin for the treatment of chronic plaque psoriasis." *European journal of dermatology : EJD* vol. 15,5 (2005): 359-62.
9. Balak, Deepak Mw, and Enes Hajdarbegovic. "Drug-induced psoriasis: clinical perspectives." *Psoriasis (Auckland, N.Z.)* vol. 7 87-94. 7 Dec. 2017, doi:10.2147/PTT.S126727
10. WebMD Medical Reference. "Drugs & Medications That Can Trigger Psoriasis Flare-Ups." *WebMD*, 7 Oct. 2020, www.webmd.com/skin-problems-and-treatments/psoriasis/drugs-worsen-psoriasis.
11. Wu, Wiggin et al. "Tonsillectomy as a treatment for psoriasis: a review." *The Journal of dermatological treatment* vol. 25,6 (2014): 482-6. doi:10.3109/09546634.2013.848258

12. Sigurdardottir, S L et al. "The association of sore throat and psoriasis might be explained by histologically distinctive tonsils and increased expression of skin-homing molecules by tonsil T cells." *Clinical and experimental immunology* vol. 174,1 (2013): 139-51. doi:10.1111/cei.12153

13. Thorleifsdottir, Ragna H et al. "Throat Infections are Associated with Exacerbation in a Substantial Proportion of Patients with Chronic Plaque Psoriasis." *Acta dermato-venereologica* vol. 96,6 (2016): 788-91. doi:10.2340/00015555-2408

14. Skudutyte-Rysstad, Rasa et al. "Association between moderate to severe psoriasis and periodontitis in a Scandinavian population." *BMC oral health* vol. 14 139. 26 Nov. 2014, doi:10.1186/1472-6831-14-139

15. Mayo Clinic Staff. "Strep Throat." *Mayo Clinic*, Mayo Foundation for Medical Education and Research, 17 Dec. 2020, www.mayoclinic.org/diseases-conditions/strep-throat/diagnosis-treatment/drc-20350344. 16. Liaw, Fang-Yih et al. "Exploring the link between cadmium and psoriasis in a nationally representative sample." *Scientific reports* vol. 7,1 1723. 11 May. 2017, doi:10.1038/s41598-017-01827-9

17. Lei, Li et al. "Abnormal Serum Copper and Zinc Levels in Patients with Psoriasis: A Meta-Analysis." *Indian journal of dermatology* vol. 64,3 (2019): 224-230. doi:10.4103/ijd.IJD_475_18

18. Barański, Marcin et al. "Higher antioxidant and lower cadmium concentrations and lower incidence of pesticide residues in organically grown crops: a systematic literature review and meta-analyses." *The British journal of nutrition* vol. 112,5 (2014): 794-811. doi:10.1017/S0007114514001366

19. Wentz, Izabella. *Hashimoto's Protocol: a 90-Day Plan for Reversing Thyroid Symptoms and Getting Your Life Back.* HarperOne, 2017.

20. Parks, Christine G et al. "Lifetime Pesticide Use and Antinuclear Antibodies in Male Farmers From the Agricultural Health Study." *Frontiers in immunology* vol. 10 1476. 11 Jul. 2019, doi:10.3389/fimmu.2019.01476

21. Parks, Christine G et al. "Insecticide use and risk of rheumatoid arthritis and systemic lupus erythematosus in the Women's Health Initiative Observational Study." *Arthritis care & research* vol. 63,2 (2011): 184-94. doi:10.1002/acr.20335

22. Yong, Wai Chung et al. "Association between Psoriasis and Helicobacter pylori Infection: A Systematic Review and Meta-analysis." *Indian journal of dermatology* vol. 63,3 (2018): 193-200. doi:10.4103/ijd.IJD_531_17

23. Neimann, Andrea L et al. "Epstein-Barr virus and human herpesvirus type 6 infection in patients with psoriasis." *European journal of dermatology : EJD* vol. 16,5 (2006): 548-52.

24. Burrows, N P et al. "A trial of oral zinc supplementation in psoriasis." *Cutis* vol. 54,2 (1994): 117-8.

25. Gupta, Mrinal et al. "Zinc therapy in dermatology: a review." *Dermatology research and practice* vol. 2014 (2014): 709152. doi:10.1155/2014/709152

26. Simonić, Edita et al. "Childhood and adulthood traumatic experiences in patients with psoriasis." *The Journal of dermatology* vol. 37,9 (2010): 793-800. doi:10.1111/j.1346-8138.2010.00870.x

27. Crosta, Maria Luigia et al. "Childhood trauma and resilience in psoriatic patients: A preliminary report." *Journal of psychosomatic research* vol. 106 (2018): 25-28. doi:10.1016/j.jpsychores.2018.01.002

A Note on "Obesity" & Weight Stigma

1. Hall, Kevin D, and Scott Kahan. "Maintenance of Lost Weight and Long-Term Management of Obesity." *The Medical clinics of North America* vol. 102,1 (2018): 183-197. doi:10.1016/j.mcna.2017.08.012

2. Schwartz, Marlene B et al. "Weight bias among health professionals specializing in obesity." *Obesity research* vol. 11,9 (2003): 1033-9. doi:10.1038/oby.2003.142

3. Devlin, Keith. "Top 10 Reasons Why The BMI Is Bogus." *National Public Radio*, 4 July 2009, www.npr.org/templates/story/story.php?storyId=106268439.

4. Firger, Jessica. "There's a Dangerous Racial Bias in the Body Mass Index." *Newsweek*, 7 May 2017, www.newsweek.com/2017/05/19/obesity-childhood-obesity-body-mass-index-bmi-weight-weight-gain-health-595625.html.

5. The Endocrine Society. "Widely Used Body Fat Measurements Overestimate Fatness In African-Americans, Study Finds." ScienceDaily. ScienceDaily, 22 June 2009. <www.sciencedaily.com/releases/2009/06/090611142407.htm>.

6. Katzmarzyk, P.T., Bray, G.A., Greenway, F.L., Johnson, W.D., Newton, R.L., Jr, Ravussin, E., Ryan, D.H. and Bouchard, C. (2011), Ethnic-Specific BMI and Waist Circumference Thresholds. Obesity, 19: 1272-1278. doi:10.1038/oby.2010.319

7. Rothman, K J. "BMI-related errors in the measurement of obesity." *International journal of obesity (2005)* vol. 32 Suppl 3 (2008): S56-9. doi:10.1038/ijo.2008.87

8. Lavie, Carl J. et al. "Obesity and Cardiovascular Diseases: Implications Regarding Fitness, Fatness, and Severity in the Obesity Paradox." Journal of the American College of Cardiology, Volume 63,

Issue 14, 2014, Pages 1345-1354, ISSN 0735-1097,
https://doi.org/10.1016/j.jacc.2014.01.022.
(http://www.sciencedirect.com/science/article/pii/S0735109714003349)
9. Shmerling, Robert H. "How Useful Is the Body Mass Index (BMI)?"
Harvard Health Blog, Harvard Medical School, 30 Mar. 2016,
www.health.harvard.edu/blog/how-useful-is-the-body-mass-index-bmi-
201603309339.
10. "Discrimination." *Healthy People 2020*, Office of Disease Prevention
and Health Promotion, www.healthypeople.gov/2020/topics-
objectives/topic/social-determinants-health/interventions-
resources/discrimination.
11. Pascoe, Elizabeth A, and Laura Smart Richman. "Perceived
discrimination and health: a meta-analytic review." *Psychological bulletin*
vol. 135,4 (2009): 531-54. doi:10.1037/a0016059
12. Alberga, A.S., Russell-Mayhew, S., von Ranson, K.M. *et al.* Weight
bias: a call to action. *J Eat Disord* 4, 34 (2016).
https://doi.org/10.1186/s40337-016-0112-4
13. Raevuori, Anu et al. "The increased risk for autoimmune diseases in
patients with eating disorders." *PloS one* vol. 9,8 e104845. 22 Aug.
2014, doi:10.1371/journal.pone.0104845
14. Hedman, Anna et al. "Bidirectional relationship between eating
disorders and autoimmune diseases." *Journal of child psychology and
psychiatry, and allied disciplines* vol. 60,7 (2019): 803-812.
doi:10.1111/jcpp.12958
15. Jenco, Melissa. "Eating Disorders Linked to Immune System
Diseases." *American Academy of Pediatrics*, 10 Nov. 2017,
www.aappublications.org/news/2017/11/10/EatingDisorders111017.
16. Kunz, Manfred et al. "Psoriasis: Obesity and Fatty Acids." *Frontiers
in immunology* vol. 10 1807. 31 Jul. 2019,
doi:10.3389/fimmu.2019.01807
17. Lee, Hansongyi et al. "Obesity, inflammation and diet." *Pediatric
gastroenterology, hepatology & nutrition* vol. 16,3 (2013): 143-52.
doi:10.5223/pghn.2013.16.3.143
18. Carrascosa, J M et al. "Obesity and psoriasis: inflammatory nature of
obesity, relationship between psoriasis and obesity, and therapeutic
implications." *Actas dermo-sifiliograficas* vol. 105,1 (2014): 31-44.
doi:10.1016/j.ad.2012.08.003
19. Yost, John, and Johann E Gudjonsson. "The role of TNF inhibitors in
psoriasis therapy: new implications for associated comorbidities." *F1000
medicine reports* vol. 1 30. 8 May. 2009, doi:10.3410/M1-30
20. Jensen, Peter, and Lone Skov. "Psoriasis and Obesity." *Dermatology
(Basel, Switzerland)* vol. 232,6 (2016): 633-639. doi:10.1159/000455840

Appendix: Resources

1. "Candida Questionnaire and Score Sheet." *The Yeast Connection*, 2003, yeastconnection.com/pdf/yeastfullsurv.pdf.
2. The EAT-26 has been reproduced with permission. Garner et al. (1982). The Eating Attitudes Test: Psychometric features and clinical correlates. Psychological Medicine, 12, 871-878
3. "Psoriasis Area and Severity Index (PASI) Worksheet." *British Association of Dermatologists*, www.bad.org.uk/shared/get-file.ashx?id=1654&itemtype=document.

ABOUT THE AUTHOR

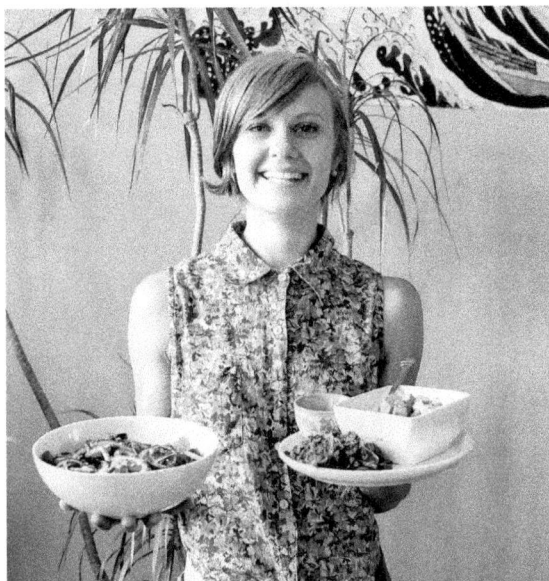

CAYLEE CLAY, RDN CDN CYT is a nationally registered and New York State certified dietitian nutritionist, certified yoga teacher, holistic researcher, food blogger, and fellow psoriasis sufferer. As a leader in the field of psoriasis and nutrition, Caylee offers a revolutionary approach to healing psoriasis. After years of researching the topic, Caylee's psoriasis is now in complete remission. Her goal is to share this powerful knowledge and help other psoriasis sufferers experience remission, too.

Caylee received her Bachelor's of Science in Nutrition and Food Studies from New York University, and completed her dietetic internship at Hunter College. Caylee has studied under industry leaders, including completing an independent study with Dr. Marion Nestle, a leading researcher in the nutrition field and author of *Food Politics*. Caylee lives in New York City with her fiance and their dog. She loves to spend her time biking around the city, shopping at farmers' markets, and gardening in her backyard.

You can learn more about Caylee by visiting her website at www.autoimmuneeats.com, following her on Instagram at @autoimmune.nutrition, and following her on Twitter at @autoimmune_eats. To schedule a one-on-one appointment to discuss your individual needs with Caylee, please visit the website and click on the "Schedule an Appointment" button.